PENGUIN BOOKS

CONQUERING ART

Suzanne Porter trained as a nurse, graduating in 1957, and has held senior appointments at various hospitals. In 1981, at the age of 45, she was diagnosed as having osteo-arthritis in her left hip joint. Within 12 months her condition had quickly deteriorated. By 1982, crippled and desperate, she began the program outlined in this book in the hope of controlling the disease. To her delight and relief, she achieved immediate success and has been in remission ever since. In 1985 Suzanne resigned from nursing to concentrate on health education and promoting the prevention of illness. She has written numerous books on the importance of diet, fitness, and maintaining a positive attitude and a healthy lifestyle; these include the best-selling cookbooks *Simply Healthy* and *It's Only Natural*. She lives in Queensland with her husband and two sons.

Suzanne Porter

CONQUERING

ARTHRITIS

*A positive program
for a healthier life*

PENGUIN BOOKS

PENGUIN BOOKS

Published by the Penguin Group
Penguin Books Australia Ltd, Ringwood, Victoria, Australia
Penguin Books Ltd, 27 Wrights Lane, London W8 5TZ, England
Penguin Books USA Inc., 375 Hudson Street, New York, New York 10014, USA
Penguin Books Canada Ltd, 10 Alcorn Avenue, Toronto, Ontario, Canada M4V 3B2
Penguin Books (NZ) Ltd, 182–190 Wairau Road, Auckland 10, New Zealand

Penguin Books Ltd, Registered Offices: Harmondsworth, Middlesex, England

First published in Australia by Viking O'Neil 1993
Published in Penguin Books 1995

10 9 8 7 6 5 4 3 2 1

Copyright © Penguin Books Australia Ltd, 1993

Typeset in Times by Midland Typesetters
Illustrations by Lorraine Ellis
Printed in Australia by Australian Print Group, Maryborough, Victoria

Acknowledgements

Thank you to my wonderful family who encouraged and supported me after I was first diagnosed, and through the years with the disease osteoarthritis.

Some of the information in this book appeared in Suzanne Porter's *Anti Arthritis Diet*. However, since that book's publication new and important evidence has emerged in the treatment of arthritis, which is now incorporated in *Conquering Arthritis*.

MY MOTTO

Never give in,
never give up,
and never retire . . .

Contents

Introduction

Unless you actually have arthritis in any of its forms, I do not believe it is possible to appreciate fully just how painful and debilitating this disease can be. Even though you are receiving all the love and support from your family and the assistance from professional care people, this is not to say these people will understand the situation fully. One of the greatest problems in the onset of the disease is the fact that although there are symptoms, there is usually no visible deformity, even after diagnosis, and therefore the victim looks perfectly normal.

From personal experience and having spoken with many people who have been diagnosed with osteo-arthritis in one or more of their joints, I have had confirmed that the pain is like a fire that never goes out in the affected joint. Even medication will barely control the pain or burning. Does this sound familiar to you? If the pain continues it has a devastating effect on the patient, causing depression and aggravating stress levels.

Osteo-arthritis affects the synovial membrane that covers the bony ends of all joints. At first it may manifest in one bone end or joint only. However, it may invade other joints as the person ages. As the disease progresses, the membrane begins to wear away and the end of the affected bone is gradually exposed. Eventually the space between the bone end narrows to such an extent that often the raw bone ends rub together, causing excruciating pain on movement.

As the disease continues to develop, the weakness in the joint becomes obvious and therefore the person may develop a noticeable limp or the hip or knee will become deformed. The sooner a corrective diet, positive thinking and meditation are adopted after diagnosis, the better are the chances of remission. I have also found through personal experience that, as long as I remain faithful to the general principles of the regime, I remain in remission. My life has changed for the better – so too can yours.

Arthritis –
a personal
approach

My story

Twelve long, wonderful years have passed since that fateful day in February 1980 when I was told by my doctor that I had osteo-arthritis in my left hip joint. The diagnosis, although not fatal, almost seemed like it at the time. The news to me was absolutely devastating and although I had nursed many people with the disease in all its stages, from early diagnosis to its most crippling, I had no idea just how painful and depressing it is. To my surprise, I was advised that the X-ray had revealed a mild degree of severity only (it was in its early stages). If that was the case, then I was even more fearful of the outcome of the disease and my general condition if and when it was at its most progressive stage!

Although I did not realise it at the time (I was too sorry for myself), it was to eventually change my life completely, giving me a new and deeper perception of people and myself. I would never be the same person again. This disease, debilitating and painful as it is, brought out in me a determination to overcome all the obstacles and adversity that such a diagnosis brings to its victims. I simply made up my mind that I would never be a cripple and I would never give in to this untimely diagnosis.

Looking back now, it seems a lifetime ago that I changed my diet from rich, fatty, oily, salty, sugary, fibre-free foods, to eating grains, vegetables and small amounts of meat (fat-free) and fruit. I remember those early days in the 80s when the first stirrings of dissatisfaction with the popular Western diet were encouraging drastic modifications. Those enlightened people who began to heed the information and facts were quickly labelled health nuts by the non-believers and one was thought of as a crank if one even dared adding bran to the diet.

In March 1981, when I first changed my diet in an effort just to be able to walk, I was subjected to much criticism and ridicule by those members of the 'health' profession with whom I worked at the time. Some were downright cruel to me and made my life hell for a time. But as I began to experience such an improvement in my condition, I quickly decided never to be intimidated by anyone where my health was concerned.

At the time, changing one's diet was held with much suspicion and scorn, but thankfully today people are more aware of the increasing evidence that the true Western diet is not the health-promoting one it was earlier thought to be. Alternatives to this diet are well and truly accepted as a natural part of daily life. But then I was the one with the disease, and knew full well just what it was like to be in such pain and unable to stand. On many an occasion in those dark days I had to drag myself along the floor to the toilet.

My books have helped hundreds of people across the world to lower blood pressure, control serum cholesterol levels, eliminate angina pain and improve arthritic conditions, among many other ailments. I now believe it is time to tell my story and encourage people with any type of disease. Don't let it beat you – be strong and determined, follow my dietary guidelines and begin using the positive thoughts and meditation detailed in a later chapter of this book. Together, they will be an added bonus to your overall health and will reduce stress levels.

Positive thinking and meditation have played a vital part in the treatment of my osteo-arthritis; their inclusion has further im-proved and expanded my life. Since I have used positive thinking and meditation, I have found I cope much better with the stresses and problems of everyday living. I now believe these valuable segments are part of the whole program for better health. Indeed, they have been recognised by health professionals as so important that they are being incorporated in the treatment of many diseases.

Today, as I write, most people are shocked when they learn I have been battling this disease for over 10 years and, to be honest, I only remember I have it if I twist my leg, which is extremely rare. To look at me, no one would ever guess. Reap the rewards of a second chance. Above all, don't be inhibited by others. It matters not what they think: you and you alone will be the one to benefit and that in itself will have a wonderful effect on both yourself and those around you.

It is my hope that this book will inspire both young and old alike to overcome any obstacles or barriers in their quest for a fitter, healthy life after diagnosis. I wish you all improved health.

What is arthritis?

The word 'arthritis' means inflammation of a joint. It is a term that relates to more than 100 different types of joint diseases. Osteo-arthritis and rheumatoid arthritis are the two most common types. Arthritis, in all its forms, is responsible for the chronic disability of millions of people, worldwide, over the age of twenty-five. It affects one person in four over the age of 65 and one person in 10 develops symptoms requiring treatment. Although a change in eating habits and lifestyle as outlined in this book will assist those with rheumatoid arthritis, it is osteo-arthritis that I am discussing in this book.

Osteo-arthritis : a definition
Osteo-arthritis affects both men and women, and can be traced back millions of years. It has been recognised in the joints of skeletons and mummies as far apart as Egypt, Peru and Africa. It is certainly not just a disease of modern-day living.

Osteo-arthritis affects mainly the weight-bearing joints, particularly the hips, knees, big toes and occasionally the neck and spine. It may develop after an injury or accident to the joint itself and, although other joints may eventually become affected, it usually affects only one. There has also been some discussion and investigation into the impact that negative thought patterns may have on the onset of arthritis. Osteo-arthritis is commonly referred to as the 'wear-and-tear disease' and, when diagnosed, may mean that you have to make changes to your lifestyle. It will certainly mean pain, stress, shock, depression and restriction of movement for most of those afflicted.

Is it curable?

The answer is no, it cannot be cured. Once the synovial membrane is damaged, the body does not seem to have the healing power to restore the membrane to its former health, regardless of treatment. However, after the initial diagnosis and medical treatment to control the inflammation is completed, it is essential that you quietly take stock of your situation and decide whether or not you are prepared to make the changes necessary to improve your condition or whether you just give in and endure the pain, discomfort, restriction and disability. Your future health and comfort are entirely in your hands.

Treatment by natural means

Unfortunately, to date, there has been little attention given to the important role that food plays in the treatment of osteo-arthritis.

Healthy joint

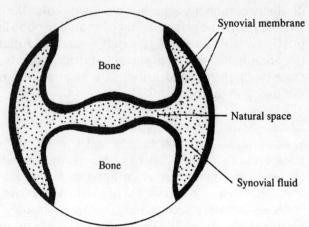

Synovial membrane

Bone

Natural space

Bone

Synovial fluid

Diseased joint

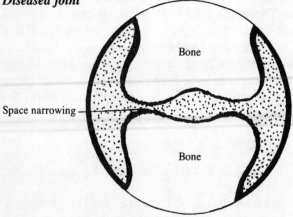

Space narrowing

Bone

Bone

Advanced stages

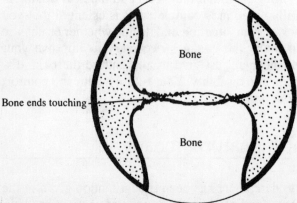

Bone ends touching

Bone

Bone

As an experienced nursing sister, it would seem to me to be one of the first areas to address, but it is the one most ignored. Why? All the scientific evidence names the fatty, oily, sugary, fibre-free Western diet as one of the major culprits in the development and exacerbation of most diseases, so surely a change of diet should be encouraged?

There are certain foods in the Western diet, for example, fatty, oily foods and sugar in all its forms, including fruit and alcohol, that create a build-up of fat in the bloodstream when eaten alone, in large quantities or collectively in the diet. This excess fat coats the red blood cells, preventing them from picking up oxygen and nutrients, which in turn creates a sludging effect, thus preventing the all-important oxygen and nutrients from being delivered to the tissues and cells, particularly depriving a diseased joint. Oxygen levels have been found to be extremely low in the joints of arthritis patients. It takes about 14 hours for excess fat to be utilised (providing, of course, no further amounts of these foods are eaten during that time) and the blood cells to return to normal function again. Imagine how the problem exacerbates as the person continues to eat a diet high in fats, oils, sugars, fruit and alcohol over a 24-hour period and what deterioration occurs to the body starved of oxygen and nutrients over a lifetime.

By adopting a diet that is centred around eating grains, vegetables and small amounts of meat (fat-free) and fruit, the blood–fat ratio begins to return to normal. I have followed these principles for just over 11 years with great success. Now 57 years of age, I take no medication, my blood pressure is normal, my cholesterol is normal and I follow a busy lifestyle.

After you have begun this program you will be pleasantly surprised at the results and you may even notice a marked improvement in your general health. You will be less stressed and begin to feel fitter and happier in your daily life.

Eating habits: a time for change?

It is said, 'You are what you eat', and 'It is never too late to change'. I am inclined to agree with both statements. But I would also add 'You are what you think'. From 18 to 80 it is never too late to change your lifestyle to improve your health. A lifetime of old eating habits may seem difficult to change – you feel comfortable, safe and happy with them – but now you have osteo-arthritis and, if you want to improve your condition, change is the direction you

will need to take. Making a conscious decision and effort to change your lifestyle will create extra bonuses:
• blood-pressure levels will drop to normal
• extra weight will disappear – you will become more agile
• cholesterol levels will drop
• blood-fat levels will drop to normal (no more red-blood-cell 'sludging')
• hypoglycaemia (low blood-sugar levels) will improve.
   Encourage the family to participate with you and support your efforts to a healthier lifestyle, particularly in the early stages of treatment. People who are alone should call on relatives and neighbours for support and help if necessary.

Weight control

It is very important to control your weight, particularly if the disease has affected the weight-bearing joints. Extra weight is an added burden to those joints already affected and may have an adverse effect. My program takes this into consideration; you will find that after several days, weight will begin to come off slowly. On the other hand, if you are not overweight and wish to maintain that weight, eat larger meals and more often.

Exercise and posture

Exercise is physical exertion for the improvement of health. When you exercise or exert yourself, you will notice an increase in the beating of your heart. This is due to the body's need for increased oxygen and nutrients to cope with the exertion. An exercise program will improve the rhythm of the heart beat and help keep the heart muscle healthy and ready for any emergency or exertion should it arise unexpectedly.
   Aerobic exercise simply means using up oxygen as you exercise. With an increase in heart rate and blood flow, more oxygen and nutrients will be delivered to all parts of the body, including the joints. Contrary to popular belief (by the lay-person), a joint does not have its own network of blood vessels; the blood is delivered and absorbed into the joints by a process known as osmosis. You may never have exercised before, but now more than ever before, because you have osteo-arthritis in your joint, you will need to include a sensible exercise program in your daily life.

It is not necessary to engage in a vigorous sport. Indeed this may aggravate your condition and cause unnecessary pain, which would be foolish. Over-exercising the affected joint may cause additional discomfort. I suggest a gentle flexing and stretching of the major joints each day, together with deep breathing exercises through the nose,* followed by a 20-minute walk. Early morning walking is best, but if that isn't possible, take a walk in the evening, or during your lunch break. Arrange to go with a family member who will keep you company and encourage you to continue, rain, hail or shine.

Don't exercise when you are sick or tired, but don't let these be an excuse to not exercise at all. Rest up if you are not feeling well. Under these circumstances practise using positive thoughts and note an improvement in your general well-being. Give some thought to the consequences before you decide to take on a strenuous activity such as sport or dancing.

There have been two occasions where I embarked on foolish activities since first I was diagnosed and changed my lifestyle. The first time was several years after I began my program. I was walking well, with no hint of the disease. I felt fit and could not resist the temptation to have a game of my beloved tennis (which I had had to give up). I played well for someone who had not played a game for several years. However, much to my sorrow, after several hours I became lame and began to limp badly. It was almost impossible to bear weight on my left leg. The pain and burning returned and for the following three days I required medication to relieve the pain and I used a walking stick. You would have thought it was enough to learn my lesson? No, two years later I danced the night away to the fast music of bush dancing. Yes, you guessed it – for the next three days I was completely bedridden and only able to drag myself to the toilet along the floor. Now I have learned my lesson and prefer to watch from the sidelines rather than go through the pain, discomfort and terror that not being able to walk can bring.

I don't recommend physiotherapy either due to personal experience. When my physiotherapist heard I had the disease, a set of hip rotation and flexing exercises were suggested to prevent muscle wasting of the affected joint. After one week of daily exercises the pain, burning, discomfort and soreness returned (at times was worse than my original pain), often lasting many hours.

* Smokers or those who have given up smoking may find nasal breathing a little difficult at first. However persevere, it won't be long before you are breathing through your nose without difficulty.

I immediately stopped those exercises and now walk or gently stretch and flex the affected joint without incurring any problems. I believe from personal experience that over-exercising can irritate the joint. Walking is really best.

Some points to take into account when exercising:
· wear well-fitting, thick-soled jogging shoes
· dress for the weather
· have a 5-minute warm-up and cool-down before and after exercising.

It is very important to stand and walk as straight as possible. Here are a few pointers I use.
· *Sitting* To avoid pressure on an affected knee or hip it is advisable to sit up straight or be well supported behind the shoulders. Always take care not to cross your legs and, where possible, elevate your feet on a padded stool. When you rise from the chair, do not move off immediately; stand up straight and allow your back and legs to be in line, taking care to allow the unaffected leg to bear most of the weight before you begin to walk.
· *Lying down* Gently make sure that your spine is straight, and if one or other of your hips is affected, take care to sit up straight and dangle your legs over the edge of the bed before you begin to rise; then place both feet flat on the floor and rise.
· *Neck or spine* If either of these is affected, wherever possible always try to keep both the neck and spine straight and well supported when sitting or standing.
· *Knees* The same principles apply as for the hips.

Avoid twisting your diseased joint, as sudden jarring may cause instant, excruciating pain and discomfort. After all these years, the only time my diseased hip is detectable is when I fail to follow the suggestions as set down here.

Osteo-arthritis, depression and anxiety

Depression and anxiety are a natural result of the diagnosis. During my nursing career, without exception, every patient I cared for with osteo-arthritis was depressed and anxious about the future and the possible changes to their lifestyle they would have to make, particularly as the disease progressed. When my diagnosis was confirmed, I was so distressed, I cried for three days, worrying about the future and the possibility that my beloved nursing career was at an end.

Hypoglycaemia (low blood sugar) with its 'highs', 'lows' and mood swings can affect those with arthritis. It is therefore very important to maintain a constant level of glucose (sugar) in the blood, thus preventing the rises and falls that alter temperament and stress levels. Eating six small meals of grains, vegetables and small amounts of meat (fat-free) and fruit each day will maintain blood-glucose (sugar) levels that are neither high nor low.

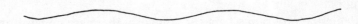

The spasmodic eating of wrong foods and missing meals will produce swings that are high and low, affecting moods and producing depression and anxiety.

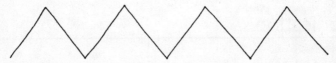

Alcohol and caffeine are stimulants that can also have an adverse affect on the nervous system, causing feelings of anxiety, depression and abnormally fast heartbeats. The dietary program I recommend will ensure that blood-glucose levels remain constant in the blood stream.

Arthritis: fallacies and facts

- *Fallacy* Osteo-arthritis is curable.
  Fact No it isn't. Once the bone ends are worn, unfortunately they are worn forever.
- *Fallacy* Diet can't possibly help me: I have eaten good food all my life.
  Fact The correct diet will help your condition: 'good' food may be foods from the fatty, oily, sugary Western diet that are not health-promoting.
- *Fallacy* I need to eat lots of fat and oil to lubricate my joints.
  Fact Neither fats nor oils are used to lubricate the joints; they require oxygen and nutrients.
- *Fallacy* Exercise will not help me at all; I have been active all my life and look at me now.
  Fact Exercise is now even more important to prevent muscle wasting, bone-density loss and increase oxygen levels.

When do I start the program?

This program has been designed for you to remain on for the rest of your life. If this prospect seems overwhelming, then look at your disease now and evaluate the consequences of remaining on the Western diet. The program has worked for me for over 10 years. I can't guarantee success for everyone, but if you don't try it for at least six weeks, you will never know if it works or not.

Begin the program whenever you wish; there are no hard-and-fast rules. However, to obtain the most benefit, I suggest you start immediately. Whether or not you go into it 'cold turkey' is up to you. You might decide to take it in small doses, get results, and gradually proceed. It is entirely up to you.

Medication

In the initial stages of the onset of the disease, it is important to work closely with your physician and follow his or her instructions implicitly. Control of pain and inflammation is imperative.

When you begin the program, you will find that your need for medication will diminish and eventually you will no longer need it. However, if the condition flares up at a later stage, seek medical advice for further medication and treatment.

I have only required medication on the two occasions mentioned earlier in this book, apart from the initial medication when I was first diagnosed (which had an adverse effect on me). If your arthritis goes into remission, after following the program, you may find the symptoms are absent or greatly diminished for quite a long time. My osteo-arthritis has been in remission for 10 years.

Remission: what is it?

Remission is a temporary abatement of a disease in a person where the disease is not evident. He or she is usually symptom-free and requires little or no medication. As I have said before, I have been in remission for the past 10 years and firmly believe I will remain in remission for many years to come.

Quackery

I mentioned earlier in this book that osteo-arthritis is incurable. Down through the ages there have been many remedies concocted as 'miracle' cures. Millions of dollars have been spent by people hoping to find a cure and solve their problems, mostly without success.

During the early part of the eighteenth century to the latter part of the last century, right through to today, it is quite common for such remedies to be peddled as 'sure-fire cures'. Wherever anyone is seeking relief from this wretched disease, someone always has a 'miracle' cure with all sorts of remedies from 'pills' and 'potions' to topical applications. I tried many approaches prior to changing my diet in an effort to relieve pain and discomfort – all to no avail. The sensible approach is with proper diet, exercise, positive thinking and meditation. Leave the quackery to others.

Osteoporosis

Osteoporosis is a bone disease whereby the bone density begins to decline due to a lack of calcium. It generally affects women during the menopause years, but it can also affect men. Poor diet, resulting from over-consumption of protein that prevents calcium being absorbed by the body and lack of exercise are the principle causes.

Don't rush to the refrigerator and consume huge amounts of foods containing calcium – it's not that easy! However, by all means eat low-fat dairy products and small amounts of protein according to my guidelines and begin to exercise. If you are in the menopause years and concerned about your calcium levels, discuss this with your physician who may recommend a calcium supplement.

Sex and osteo-arthritis

I have mentioned the adoption, after diagnosis, of a particular diet, exercise program, positive thinking, meditation and many other factors, but now I must discuss the very important subject of how to cope with sexual activity. Has all sexual activity ceased for you since you were diagnosed? I hope not. This very delicate, personal and intimate subject is rarely discussed or approached. I can't understand why: perhaps because osteo-arthritis affects people who are mostly over 65 and it is considered that they no longer enjoy this activity?

It is an important subject and, curiously, one that is rarely acknowledged by those in the health profession or by counsellors. Has anyone ever discussed it with you since you were diagnosed? In all the literature I have read over the years, without exception, no one ever mentions how to cope with this sensitive subject, or what measures need to be adopted in order to continue an active sex life after diagnosis. Don't be afraid to discuss with your partner any problems or difficulties that might arise, particularly if the disease affects either one or both hip joints. Your partner will need to have a special understanding of your condition and a sensitive approach. Seek the advice of a counsellor who is well versed in sexual matters and who will guide you both with new techniques and positions. There may be times, too, when you have pain and discomfort and sexual activity is a 'no no'. Your partner should be of assistance and support during these difficult but, one hopes, short periods. With a little thought, sexual activity can still be an exciting and fulfilling activity.

Breaking the diet: is it worth it?

Because the Western diet is so tempting, there will always be a tendency to slip back and indulge in former eating habits. Naturally, you will be very keen and disciplined at first when you begin the program, but your body will take a little time to adjust to the elimination of fats, oils and sugary foods, so be patient; on the other hand, you might find you are feeling so much better and those former foods no longer tempt you. You may find, however, occasions such as birthdays, weddings, anniversaries and festive occasions that will require a little forethought on your part as to how to deal with them. Don't become apprehensive about how to cope with the menu when the time comes. If it is impossible to resist the food selection, follow any one of these tips.

- Wherever possible be firm with yourself and remain faithful to the program. Take some of the 'program food' along with you.
- Discuss your position with your hosts, who will certainly be sympathetic to your needs.
- Resist the urge to eat gravy and skin on your meat. Trim off any fat and bypass the heavy dessert; instead order fruit salad, without any topping.

- Go off the program just this once and enjoy it, without feeling guilty. However, be prepared for the possible return of pain and discomfort. Decide whether or not it is worth it.
- Eat everything in sight. Enjoy the occasion but don't complain when the pain and discomfort return.

After several years on the program (yes, it is for life!) you might discover you can occasionally eat foods that used to affect you before you began the program, particularly if you are also adopting the positive thoughts and meditation. However, be cautious and selective. Returning to your former bad dietary habits may affect your general health. For example, your cholesterol levels and blood pressure may become elevated.

Being positive

In the two years since I wrote *The Anti Arthritis Diet* more evidence has emerged supporting the need to include positive thinking in the treatment of arthritis, particularly in the control of pain. Negative thoughts, feelings and actions are a total waste of time and energy. They do not achieve anything, except to have a negative effect on the person, which in turn is debilitating. Curiously, most people who develop arthritis are usually highly critical of themselves and other people. They set incredibly high standards and expectations both for themselves and others, often demanding perfection that is unrealistic and impossible to meet.

I was a perfect example of this until I realised that in order to help my condition I needed both a dietary program and a more positive outlook on life. It is now more than ever necessary to change your way of thinking. Accentuate the positive, eliminate the negative. Exchange your negative thoughts for powerful positive ones and reap the rewards of a much happier, healthier you. It will have a positive effect on those around you.

I have listed below 31 powerful patterns or affirmations for you to use, one for every day of one month. They have been created to help you rid yourself of those old out-of-date negative ones.

How to use the thoughts or affirmations

Begin with number one and repeat it to yourself at least 100 times during the first day. Set aside some time during the day to write it out at least 20 times. The following day select the second one and so on until you have completed these sayings or affirmations for one month. You will be amazed at just how positive you will become and how others will respond positively to you. When you have completed the month, you may wish to commence the entire program for another month and so on until the thoughts are a part of your daily life.

1 There is no room in my life for negative thoughts.
2 I have the power to bring about change in my life.
3 I am learning to love myself.
4 By changing myself, I become powerful.
5 There is no room in my life for critical thoughts.
6 I have the power to bring about change by my thoughts.
7 I am no longer angry or tense. I am at peace with myself.
8 There is no room in my life for the word hate.
9 It is a beautiful day and I love the world (even when it's raining).
10 I believe in myself today, tomorrow and always.
11 I radiate love and positive thinking.
12 By accepting myself with love, I am open to forgive.
13 I strive to be that which I want to be.
14 My thoughts are powerful and strong.
15 I radiate love and happiness.
16 I am creating harmony at all times.
17 I choose to be healthy and prosperous.
18 I have confidence in myself at all times.
19 Criticism is all-consuming: I will leave it to others.
20 I am willing to create new successes for myself.
21 I feel happy with myself. I am whole again.
22 I am peaceful at all times.
23 I am a happy, successful person.
24 Today I climb the mountain and walk tall.
25 I forgive myself and forgive others.
26 I am free to leave anger and hate behind me.
27 I am centred in my life and my life is good.
28 Through love, wisdom and peace I achieve all I desire.
29 I choose to be healthy at all times.
30 I am free of criticism.
31 I am a beautiful, loving person.

Meditation

Much has been said about meditation and often the value of taking time out to meditate for oneself is looked upon with scorn and scepticism. Indeed, most of us were brought up to disregard our importance in favour of unselfishly doing for others. To such an extent was this instilled into our heads that even today precious little time is afforded the self. I cannot stress too seriously the importance of meditation and the power it has to improve the health of those who regularly practise it.

Most people will quickly say that they do not have any time during the day in which to meditate; however, with a little thought and preparation, one can always set aside some time during the 24 hours of the day. There is nothing wrong with meditating just after retiring to bed when it is peaceful and quiet or perhaps in the office during the lunch break!

How to meditate

If possible have a tape-recorder playing soft, peaceful music or, if that is not practicable, meditate without. Select an area where it is relatively quiet and, with shoes off, either sit up straight in a chair with the feet flat on the floor or lie down flat on the floor. Close your eyes and allow your arms to rest lightly on your thighs with the tip of each index finger touching the tip of each thumb, making a circle, with the other fingers extended. Breathe quietly in and out through the nostrils (mouth closed), repeat the following affirmation as you breathe in, and repeat it again as you breathe out.

I am that I am (in), I am that I am (out).

Continue to repeat the saying while you meditate, allowing no other thoughts in your head other than the words you are repeating quietly while maintaining the breathing technique. If you find other thoughts are creeping into your mind, don't become irritated or angry; just allow them to pass through and continue on as in-structed. When you have concluded the meditation, very quietly and slowly open your eyes and return to your surroundings. You will be surprised how relaxed and free from tension you feel on completion of the meditation.

Combining the program with positive thoughts and meditation will greatly improve your outlook on life. For better health, I believe it is necessary to incorporate all these elements – diet, exercise, positive thoughts and meditation – and that they are inexorably linked.

The diet

This diet takes into consideration the importance of good nutrition for better health and ensures your body has the right fuel. If, however, you are concerned that the essential nutrients are missing from your food source, I suggest you take a multivitamin and mineral tablet. You might like to discuss this with your physician. This program is high in the consumption of complex carbohydrates (starches) and dietary fibre and low in simple carbohydrates (sugars), meat and fruit, with no added fats, oils or sugar. Alcohol is limited to cooking only and smoking is discouraged.

Food sensitivities

There may be many foods to which you are sensitive, even before diagnosis; this, however, is an individual condition. Food that may be OK for one person may have an adverse effect on another and so on. Wherever possible, select fresh and processed foods that are free from chemicals, artificial flavourings, colourings and additives. Carefully read all labels. Look for fat, oil, salt and sugar content and if in doubt about any ingredient don't include it on your shopping list.

There is a family of foods that many people believe has an adverse effect on arthritics. These foods are known as the 'nightshade' vegetables and I suggest before you listen to the information regarding these foods, try each one of them separately to ascertain if they have adverse effect on you. Denying them without trial could mean overlooking the fact that you are not sensitive to any of them; therefore you might be missing out on the pleasure they could give you.

- *Potatoes* Includes all varieties. Eat both the skin and flesh. However, don't eat them if the skin has turned green.
- *Tomatoes* Includes all shapes, colours and varieties.
- *Eggplant* Includes both small and large.
- *Capsicum* These come in several colours – red, green, yellow and purple – and range from mild to hot.

If after eating any of the above foods you have pain or stiffness (either immediately or over the next 24 hours), then it would be advisable to cross it off your shopping list. Remember, we are all individuals and each of us reacts differently.

I have completed the 'nightshade' test and found that only tomatoes, when consumed in large amounts, affect me. If I eat them in small amounts I am fine. As a trial, I also eliminated potatoes from my diet for three months about six years ago, and I found out that they do not affect me. This is a blessing, as I love potatoes! They are a great standby but lots of willpower is needed to refrain from adding sour cream or herb butter, which are a 'no no'.

Finding out if you are sensitive to foods can only be accomplished by trial and error. I suggest you fill out a diary, and each day for a month write down everything you eat: what it was; the time; why you ate it and any after-effects such as pain, stiffness, discomfort and so on. It may sound tedious, but make it into a game and you will soon discover the advantages of knowing to which foods you do or don't react. This way you will know what to buy each week when shopping. Some suggest that over-consumption of grains, breads and cereals have an adverse effect on everyone suffering from arthritis. Again, experiment and evaluate any effect. These foods have never affected me adversely.

'Go' foods

The following foods are on your 'go' list. You may eat these as desired, unless of course you have tested sensitive to any of them. The list is by no means complete; however, it does give a large range from which to choose.

Complex carbohydrates (starches), in the form of grains and vegetables, make up about 80 per cent of the total kilojoules/calories you require and may be eaten in unlimited amounts.

Breads may be eaten on this program. However, the approved breads recommended contain no added fats, oils or sugar. Examples include Pritikin bread and rolls, sourdough breads, rye breads, flat breads such as mountain, Lebanese or pita, or scones as given in the recipes in this book (see pp. 97, 98).

Dietary fibre is the non-digestible part of all plant foods. It is essential to all diets and prevents constipation. This program and the recipes in this book are high in dietary fibre. You may also add extra fibre from wheat (unprocessed bran), oats (oatbran), rice (ricebran granules) and barley (bran).

Vegetables

artichokes, globe and Jerusalem
asparagus
beans, runner and snap, all colours
beetroot
Brussels sprouts
cabbage, all colours
capsicum, all colours
carrots
cauliflower
celery
chives, plain and garlic
corn
cucumber
eggplant
endive
fennel
garlic
leeks
lettuce, all colours
mushrooms, all varieties including dried
onions, Spanish, brown, white and salad
parsnips
peas, snap, snow and sugar
potatoes, including sweet potatoes
pumpkin
radishes
silverbeet
spinach
sprouted grains and seeds (all varieties)
swede
tomatoes, all varieties including yellow and green
turnip
zucchini

Grains

This includes: whole, flakes, steel-cut or flour (preferably stoneground)

arrowroot
barley
bulghur
cornflour
flour*:buckwheat, rye,
triticale, unbleached white, wholemeal, barley
millet
rice, white, brown, wild or mixed

Pasta (egg-yolk-free)

buckwheat
cannelloni, instant tubes
lasagne, instant sheets
macaroni
spaghetti

* Plain (all-purpose) flour. When self-raising flour is used as an ingredient in a recipe, it will be stated.

Breads

mountain bread
pancakes, crêpes, scones
pita, wholegrain
rye bread made from
   sourdough

rye crisps, no added fats, oils
   or sugar
wholemeal (approved, see
   p. 24), no added fats, oils or
   sugar

Cereals

grapenuts cereal
puffed cereals
puffed wheat
rice, cooked, all varieties

rolled oats, wheat, barley and
   rye
vita-brits
weeties

Lentils and pulses

Although high in protein, these are filling, satisfying and an excellent replacement for meat. If eaten in very large quantities, this food comes under the 'caution' list. One serving (1½ cups cooked pulses) per meal is recommended.

black-eyed peas
blue boiling peas
broad beans, fresh or dried
calico beans
chickpeas
haricot beans

lentils, brown, green and red
lima beans
navy beans
red kidney beans
split peas, yellow and green

Eggs

whites only (discard yolks)

'Caution' foods

The following list gives some of the key foods you will now be incorporating in your program. If eaten in excess, these foods may cause blood-fat levels to rise. Where necessary I have given serving sizes.

Eat proteins in the form of animal meats (fat-free), and dried beans, dried peas and lentils (see under 'Go' foods). Eat 1 × 100 g/ 3½ oz meat every seven days for the first month. Then gradually increase your meat intake to about four or five times (same size serving). This will make up about 10–15 per cent of the total kilojoules/calories that you require.

Drink decaffeinated tea and decaffeinated coffee very sparingly. Wherever practical, use herb teas and coffee substitutes.

Added salt has been listed under the caution foods. If you do not have elevated blood-pressure levels I recommend the use of low-salt soy sauce. Although a diet high in fats and oils is the main contributor to high blood pressure, salt is still regarded by many health professionals as the main culprit; it is therefore definitely not permitted.

However, I have used my program with many people, including a five-week one with volunteers, and those with elevated blood-pressure levels found a return to normal levels after only three weeks when they eliminated fats and oils, even though they were allowed to use low-salt soy sauce. Low-salt soy sauce is therefore an option in all my savoury recipes. Do not, however, add salt to cooking and remember that added salt causes the body to retain excess water. The decision to refrain from adding salt to your food should be discussed with your physician and is a matter of personal choice.

Fresh fruit is full of fibre and has differing amounts of fruit sugar (fructose), depending on the ripeness of each piece. Fruit is used in small amounts each day and may be fresh or cooked in natural juice without added sugar. Limit your intake to about five pieces per day, particularly in the early stages. You may find that with a regular exercise program, blood sludging is no longer present and therefore you can eat extra.

Fruit*

apples, all varieties and colours	mandarins
apricots	mangoes
bananas	nectarines
blackberries	oranges
blueberries	papaw
cantaloup	passionfruit
cherries	peaches
figs	pears
gooseberries	pineapple
grapefruit	plums
grapes, all colours	raspberries
guava	rhubarb
honeydew melon	rockmelon
kiwi fruit	strawberries
lemons	tangellos
lychees	watermelon

* No more than three to five pieces per day.

Dairy
cottage cheese, non-fat,
 uncreamed
skim milk, 1 cup per day
skim-milk powder, used as
 part of daily allowance

skim milk, canned, evaporated,
 used as part of daily
 allowance
yoghurt, non-fat, sugar-free

Meats
beef
chicken
lamb
pork

rabbit
turkey
veal

Fish and seafood
crayfish
fish, low-fat varieties
lobster
prawns

salmon, canned, water-packed
scallops
shrimp
tuna, canned, water-packed

'Stop' foods

On this program the total fat and oil intake needs to be between 5 and 10 per cent of the total kilojoule/calorie intake. This will be derived from the fat or oil naturally present in the food we eat, which includes grains, vegetables, fruits and non-fat dairy products. Adding processed fats and oils to either cooked or raw foods will contribute another 10–15 per cent above the intake required.

Foods not recommended are as follows.
- added fats or oils including butter, margarine and fatty spreads
- avocado, olives and nuts (all too high in natural fats or oils)
- egg yolks
- caffeine beverages, soft drinks and sugar-sweetened fruit drinks
- all cakes, puddings, biscuits and scones made with fat or oil, sugar, salt and egg yolks (either home-made or commercial)
- whole milk, cream, mayonnaise, fatty cheese and fatty yoghurt
- meat spreads and meats (when eaten in larger quantities than those specified in the list of 'caution' foods), bacon, ham or sausages
- all dressings, sauces, spreads and toppings made with fat or oil, salt, sugar (either home-made or commercial)
- all foods fried in fat or oil regardless of type and brand

- nuts, or oils from nuts and vegetables (with the exception of chestnuts)
- alcohol, except in cooking
- home-made or commercial jams or jellies made with fats or oils, salt or sugar

  These 'stop' foods may be eaten in small quantities only. Stop and think before including them in your program.

Dried fruit

Daily maximum is 50 g/2 oz unless blood-fat levels are normal. Where possible buy natural, sun-dried and unsulphured fruits.

apples	mango
apricots	peach
bananas	pear
currants	pineapple, crystallised (wash
dates	off sugar)
figs	raisins
ginger, crystallised (wash off	sultanas
sugar)	

Alcohol

Use sparingly in cooking to enhance the flavour.

brandy .	rum
dry white wine	sherry
red wine	whisky

Daily menu

The following menu has been created as a guide to what foods you can eat. It allows for six meals per day including supper and takes into consideration those with a healthy appetite. However, if you have a weight problem and losing a few kilograms/pounds is necessary, then all you need do is cut down on the size of the meal or perhaps eliminate supper. If on the other hand you are trying to maintain your weight, then all you need do is increase the size of your servings.

Breakfast
cereal, large serve (see p. 26 for choices)
skim milk
fresh fruit
2 slices toast (approved, see p. 24)
fruit spread (sugar-free)
beverage (see p. 26 for choices)

or

cooked vegetables
piece of citrus fruit
beverage as above

Morning tea
piece of fruit or muffin (see p. 96)
beverage as above

Lunch
soup (see pp. 39–45 for choices) or sandwich (approved, see p. 24)
small salad (see pp. 46–52 for choices)
piece of fruit
beverage as above

Afternoon tea
2–4 dry biscuits (see p. 26 for choices)
fruit spread of choice (sugar-free)
beverage as above

Dinner
Crispy Baked Potato Shells (see p. 54)
meat as per guidelines or vegetable main meal, large serve (see
    pp. 53–68 for choices)
3 differently coloured vegetables, steamed (see p. 25 for choices)
dessert or pudding, hot or cold (see pp. 86–95 for choices)
beverage as above

Supper
sandwich using approved bread (see p. 24), fresh or toasted (see
    p. 69 for choices)
piece of fruit or muffin (see p. 96)
beverage as above

Planning ahead

Many cooks, both male and female, work outside the home, often holding down a job as well as running a busy home and caring for a family. Working out menus, shopping for ingredients and preparing meals require skilled planning. Here are some suggestions.

- For each week sit down and select meals for the entire family. Make a list of all ingredients necessary to service each menu. This will save precious time, and is an economical way to run a busy kitchen.
- Shop once per week when the food supplies are at their freshest and the store is the least busy. Where practical, grow your own vegetables.
- Meals can be made up in advance and refrigerated or frozen for later use. I suggest you make double the quantity of a recipe, use half and flavour the remainder with garlic or curry powder. Freeze this second half for later use. Salad vegetables can be washed, drained and made up an hour or so before using and refrigerated. Where a dressing is recommended, add this just prior to serving, unless it will not spoil the salad if added earlier.

Cooking with flair

With a little flair and imagination you will produce some excellent meals. You will be surprised just how colourful, appetising and tasty they will be. The whole family will want to be on your program. From tangy sauces to superb soups, the recipes in this book are for everyday use. Experiment with herbs and spices for added flavour and zing. However, take care not to overdo it at first, but gradually increase the amounts to enhance the flavour of your food. It is very easy to spoil a recipe by spicing too heavily.

Wherever possible and practical use fresh instead of dried herbs. Remember to add them during the last 20 minutes of cooking. Include herbs in soups, sauces, breads, scones and in all types of savoury recipes, particularly where no added salt is used.

Herbs
Anise seed, aniseed may be used in breads and scones. The seeds may be crushed. It has a subtle licorice flavour.
Basil Sweet basil is wonderful with tomatoes and potatoes. Use in soups, salads, juices and meat or vegetable casseroles and stews.
Bay leaves are delicately flavoured and come from a large Mediterranean tree. They are used in soups, meat or vegetable casseroles, and vegetable and tomato juices. Remove the leaves after cooking and before serving.
Caraway seeds have a strong, sweetish flavour. They are often used in rye breads, and also with cabbage, low-fat cheeses, scones, cakes and savoury recipes. Crush before adding to salads and vegetables.
Celery seeds have a very strong flavour. Use sparingly in pickles, relishes and potato salad.
Chervil is a type of parsley and is used to flavour soups, cheese, spinach and mornays.
Chives come in plain or garlic varieties. Use in low-fat cheeses, soups, casseroles, potatoes and as a garnish (usually snipped) over salads, potatoes and spaghetti.
Coriander is used as seed or ground. Add to breads, scones, pumpkin and potato salad.
Dill has very delicate leaves with a strong flavour. Use either seed or weed with cabbage, cucumber, and in vegetable soups, low-fat cottage cheese and non-fat yoghurt. It is often used as a garnish.
Garlic may be used fresh, in powder and as granules. Add to all manner of savoury recipes: salads, soups, sauces and dressings.

Herbs

Horseradish is a white, extremely hot taproot from the mustard family that has been used for centuries. Use grated to enhance sauces and dressings.

Marjoram is a beautifully flavoured member of the mint family. It is used fresh or as dried flakes to flavour meats, mushrooms, rice, stews and casseroles, and as a garnish and flavour to vegetarian meals. Combine with parsley, chervil and thyme.

Mint leaves, from the Mentha family, are used fresh or as dried flakes to flavour salads, potatoes, peas, fruit drinks and as a garnish.

Oregano has a very strong pungent odour. Use fresh or dried in Mexican and Italian recipes, and with tomatoes, potatoes, breads, zucchini, chilli and bean recipes.

Parsley is widely known and used. Its lovely green foliage adds colour as a garnish. It is often used in white sauces, soups, casseroles and meat stews.

Poppy seeds are used as a topping on breads, cakes and slices and to garnish rice and salads.

Rosemary is added to stuffings, breads and scones; it is also used with spinach, peas, corn and cauliflower and lamb recipes. Use sprigs or dried.

Sage has a spicy flavour and has been used in Asian cooking for centuries. It is excellent for stuffings, soups, tomatoes, potatoes and rice.

Sesame seeds may be fresh or toasted. They add flavour and colour to breads, salads, cakes and muffins.

Sorrel has small spinach-like leaves. Use in soups, salads and stews.

(continued over)

Herbs *(continued)*

Tarragon has a unique flavour and is often used to flavour vinegars. Use in sauces, salads, dressings, and with tomatoes, onions and mushrooms.

Thyme has dainty small leaves with a strong flavour. Use in a bouquet garni. It is a superb addition to soups, meats, breads, stuffings and chowders, and gives flavour to peas, onions, beans and carrots.

Spices

Liberal use of spices according to taste will enhance savoury and sweet dishes alike. Buy them packaged whole, flaked or powdered.

Some spices in common use are given below.

Allspice has a strong flavour. Use in fruit cakes, slices and desserts.

Cinnamon is a delicate, powdered spice. Use in cakes, desserts, in apple recipes and as a dusting on top of cakes and in some skim-milk drinks and smoothies.

Cloves are used whole or powdered. They add that delicate flavour to apples and apple desserts (if whole, remove before eating). Add grated to enhance the flavour of fruit cakes and puddings, pickles and chutneys.

Curry powder is a combination of several spices. Its universal use to enhance the flavour of Indian dishes is well accepted. Use in curries, stews, breadings, casseroles, chutneys, Mexican and chilli bean recipes.

Ginger is freshly grated or powdered. Use in salads, fruit cakes and puddings, and in chutneys, relishes, salads, stews, casseroles, soups, vegetarian and Chinese recipes.

Mustard, dry Use in breadings, dressings, pickles, chutneys and relishes.

Spices

Nutmeg is freshly grated or bought from a store, grated. This delicate spice is added to fruit cakes and desserts, and is used with skim-milk custards and as a topping on skim-milk drinks and smoothies.

Some cooking terms

au gratin A white-sauced vegetable topped with cheese and baked in the oven.
bake Cooking by dry heat in an oven.
blanch Immerse the food for several minutes in boiling water.
blend Mix together two or more ingredients.
boil Heating until mixture begins to bubble.
chill Refrigerate until cold.
garnish The use of certain foods to decorate a completed dish, such as parsley, mint, chives, fruit, cherries, herbs (in sprigs – whole or chopped) and carved raw foods.
non-stick Means a surface that has been coated with a substance to prevent the food from sticking to it. This eliminates the need to use fats or oils as a coating.
pre-heat Turning on the oven to heat it to the required temperature before cooking the food.
purée Using a sieve, blender or processor to produce a thick liquid.
sauté To toss food, lightly turning it as it cooks; within the context of this book, oil is not used. In some recipes the instruction calls for sautéing with the pan covered; this preserves the moisture in the food, thus preventing burning.
season Add flavours of choice, for example, herbs and spices.
simmer Gently cook over a low heat just below boiling point.
steam Food cooked in a perforated container over a pot of boiling water.
stew Slowly cooking food in liquid for a long time. Often used to render cheap cuts of meat tender.
toast To brown food (usually seeds) in a pan or oven for variety and colour. Bread and cake crumbs are also treated this way.
toss Mix together a collection of different foods, usually salads or vegetables or meat to be coated in flour or other covering.
whip Rapidly beat to add air, as in stiffly beaten egg white.

*T*he recipes

The following recipes provide tasty, nutritious and satisfying meals that will support your program. They include foods drawn mainly from the 'go' and 'caution' lists given on pages 24–8; recipes that include meats and seafoods use these ingredients in small amounts only to remain within the guidelines of the program. Experiment with the ingredients and make up your own recipes as you become more familiar with the diet.

Soups

Broccoli and potato soup

SERVES 4

2 heads broccoli, chopped
2 large potatoes, chopped
1 large onion, chopped
6 cups water or defatted stock
½ tablespoon low-salt soy sauce (optional)
1 tablespoon grated parmesan cheese
generous pinch cayenne pepper
snipped chives for garnishing

Place the broccoli, potatoes, onions and liquid in a large saucepan.
Bring to the boil and simmer uncovered until vegetables are tender.
Purée in a blender until smooth. Return to saucepan. Add remaining ingredients and heat through. Garnish with chives.

Chilled papaw soup

SERVES 4

1 large papaw
2 cups fresh orange juice
1 tablespoon orange liqueur (optional)
1 tablespoon grated orange rind
fine strips orange rind (pith removed) for garnishing

Seed the papaw. Purée in a blender until smooth. Add remaining ingredients. Chill and serve garnished with orange rind.

VARIATION

Add 1 slice fresh pineapple and 1 small mango, sliced, to the papaw before blending.

Corn and chicken chowder

SERVES 4

1 cup chopped cooked chicken
2½–3 cups corn kernels
3 small potatoes, chopped
1 carrot, diced
4 cups water
4 tablespoons skim-milk powder
1 tablespoon cornflour mixed with a little water
½ tablespoon low-salt soy sauce (optional)
generous pinch cayenne pepper

Remove fat and skin from chicken. Place the vegetables and water in a large saucepan. Bring to the boil uncovered and gently simmer for about 25 minutes until vegetables are tender. Add remaining ingredients and gently simmer for a further 15 minutes until soup is thick.

Country-style red bean soup

SERVES 4

1½ cups drained canned red kidney beans
4 tomatoes, peeled and chopped
2 onions, finely chopped
2 cloves garlic, minced
4 cups water
1 tablespoon low-salt soy sauce (optional)
1 tablespoon chopped parsley
1 teaspoon dried thyme
1 bay leaf
pinch cayenne pepper

Soak the red kidney beans in fresh water for 1 hour, then drain. Place all ingredients except the beans in a large saucepan, leaving the lid off. Bring to the boil and gently simmer for about 30 minutes. Add beans and simmer for a further 15 minutes. Remove bay leaf and serve.

Cream of lentil soup

SERVES 4

1 cup lentils of choice or mixed
1 carrot, grated
1 onion, chopped
6 whole cloves
5 cups defatted stock
½ cup dry sherry or water
4 tablespoons skim-milk powder
2 tablespoons grated lemon peel
1 tablespoon low-salt soy sauce (optional)
pinch cayenne pepper

Place lentils, carrot, onions, cloves and stock in a large saucepan. Bring to the boil and gently simmer, uncovered, for about 1 hour, until lentils are tender. Add remaining ingredients, simmer for a further 5 minutes. Remove cloves and serve.

Curried zucchini and tomato soup

SERVES 4

4 large zucchini, chopped
1 large onion, chopped
1 small potato, chopped
1 clove garlic, crushed
4 cups defatted stock
2 tablespoons salt-free tomato paste
1 tablespoon skim-milk powder
1 tablespoon low-salt soy sauce (optional)
3 teaspoons curry powder
pinch powdered ginger
pinch cayenne pepper

Place zucchini, onion, potato, garlic and defatted stock in a large saucepan. Bring to the boil and gently simmer uncovered until vegetables are tender. Purée in a blender and return to saucepan. Add remaining ingredients and serve.

Fruity prune soup

SERVES 4

3 cups chopped pitted prunes
¼ cup sultanas
4 cups water
1 cinnamon stick
grated rind ½ orange
grated rind ½ lemon

Soak prunes and sultanas in the water overnight. Next day place
all ingredients in a large saucepan and gently simmer uncovered
for about 15 minutes. Discard cinnamon stick. Cool and purée in
a blender until smooth. Chill and serve.

Hazel's tomato vegetable chowder

SERVES 4

3 tomatoes, chopped
4 potatoes, chopped
1 cup peas
1 onion, chopped
4 cups defatted chicken stock
1 tablespoon low-salt soy sauce (optional)
1 tablespoon cornflour mixed with a little water
1 teaspoon apple juice concentrate
½ teaspoon garlic powder
¼ teaspoon powdered ginger
pinch cayenne pepper

Place tomatoes, potatoes, peas, onion and defatted stock in a large
saucepan. Bring to the boil and gently simmer uncovered until
tender. Add remaining ingredients and simmer for a further
15 minutes until thick.

VARIATION

Add 3 tablespoons skim-milk powder together with the soy sauce,
cornflour, apple juice concentrate and seasonings.

Quick tomato soup

SERVES 4

2 cups salt-free tomato paste
1½ cups water
½ cup canned evaporated skim milk
1 teaspoon apple juice concentrate
1 teaspoon low-salt soy sauce (optional)
½ teaspoon garlic powder
¼ teaspoon mixed spice
¼ teaspoon onion powder
pinch cayenne pepper
extra water if necessary

Thoroughly mix tomato paste and water in a large saucepan. Add
remaining ingredients. Stir well and gently simmer uncovered until
hot. Add extra water if too thick.

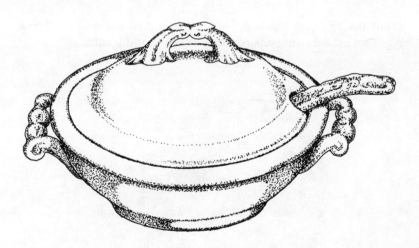

Southern soup

SERVES 4

1 carrot, grated
1 cup cooked chicken with fat and skin removed
4–6 cups chopped pumpkin
1½ cups chopped sweet potato
1 onion, chopped
4 cups defatted chicken stock
1 tablespoon low-salt soy sauce (optional)
¼ teaspoon nutmeg
¼ teaspoon garlic powder
pinch cayenne pepper

Save ½ cup grated carrot for garnishing. Place chicken, pumpkin,
sweet potato, onion, remaining grated carrot and defatted stock
in a large saucepan. Bring to the boil and gently simmer uncovered
until vegetables are tender. Add remaining ingredients and simmer
for a further 10 minutes. Serve garnished with the grated carrot.

VARIATION

Omit the chicken and add 1–1½ cups mixed seafood of choice,
e.g. fish, prawns, mussels, shrimp, scallops and lobster.

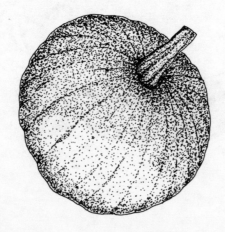

Winter vegetable soup

SERVES 4-6

1 cup chopped cauliflower
1 turnip, chopped
1 small swede, chopped
1 potato, diced
1 small carrot, diced
½ cup fresh or frozen corn kernels
1 tablespoon barley
6 cups water or defatted stock
½ cup mixed sprouted grains or seeds
1 tablespoon low-salt soy sauce (optional)
pinch garlic powder
pinch cayenne pepper

Place cauliflower, turnip, swede, potato, carrot, corn, barley and liquid in a large saucepan. Bring to the boil and gently simmer uncovered for about 1 hour or until the barley is cooked. Add remaining ingredients about 10 minutes before serving.

Salads

Apple and bean salad

SERVES 4-6

1 cup drained canned 3-bean mix
1 red apple, cored and chopped
1 green apple, cored and chopped
1 cup chopped celery
1 salad onion, chopped
1 tablespoon snipped chives
2 tablespoons lemon juice
1 cup Sweet Dressing (see p. 112)

Soak the beans in fresh water for 1 hour and drain. Toss apples in lemon juice. Carefully combine the ingredients, taking care not to damage the beans. Chill and serve.

VARIATION

Add 1 cup mixed, cooked rice to the above ingredients.

Beetroot salad delight

SERVES 4

1 beetroot
1 × 400 g/14 oz can artichoke hearts
1 small salad onion, sliced into rings
1 cup alfalfa sprouts
2 tablespoons snipped chives
1 cup Fruity Dressing (see p. 106)
1 tablespoon toasted sesame seeds for garnishing

Cook, cool, skin and slice the beetroot. Drain and quarter the artichoke hearts. Then arrange alfalfa sprouts on a round, flat dish. Carefully arrange remaining ingredients on top of the sprouts and pour the dressing over this. Sprinkle with toasted sesame seeds.

Cabbage, apple and prune salad

SERVES 4-6

2 cups finely sliced green cabbage
½ cup finely sliced red cabbage
1 red apple, cored and grated
8–10 soft prunes, pitted
1 cup Tangy Yoghurt Dressing (see p. 113)

Carefully combine all ingredients. Turn into a glass salad bowl. Chill and serve.

Cottage cheese salad

SERVES 4

1 cup non-fat, salt-free cottage cheese
4 mignonette lettuce cups
1 apple, cored and thinly sliced
4 fresh or canned unsweetened pineapple rings, halved
1 stalk celery, finely diced
½ cup Sweet Dressing (see p. 112)

Divide cottage cheese into 4 equal portions and place one in each lettuce cup. Toss together apple, pineapple and celery and then spoon over cottage cheese. Top with dressing just prior to serving.

Chickpea salad

SERVES 4

1 cup drained chickpeas
2 cups endive pieces (bite-size)
1 small salad onion, finely diced
10 cherry tomatoes, halved
½ cup Orange Soy Dressing (see p. 110)

Carefully toss all ingredients and arrange in a small glass salad bowl. Chill and serve.

Cucumber salad with green dressing

SERVES 4-6

3 cucumbers, peeled and sliced
1 small salad onion, finely diced
1¼ cups Green Dressing (see p. 106)

Arrange cucumber in a small glass salad bowl. Combine salad onion with dressing and pour over cucumbers. Chill and serve.

Fresh beetroot special

SERVES 4-6

2 raw beetroots, peeled and grated
1 large green apple, cored and grated
2 tablespoons snipped chives
½ cup Orange Soy Dressing (see p. 110)

Carefully combine all ingredients. Chill and serve.

Fruit 'n' chicken salad

SERVES 4

1 cup chopped cooked chicken
1 apple, cored and chopped
2 canned unsweetened peach halves, sliced
1 stalk celery, diced
2 tablespoons snipped chives
4 lettuce cups
1 cup Strawberry Dressing (see p. 112)

Remove fat and skin from chicken. Carefully combine chicken, apple, peaches, celery and chives. Divide into 4 equal portions and spoon one into each lettuce cup. Spoon Strawberry Dressing over the salad just prior to serving.

VARIATION

Replace the chicken with 8 king prawns, cooked, shelled, deveined and chopped.

Fruity coleslaw

SERVES 4-6

½ green cabbage, finely sliced
1 salad onion, finely chopped
1 small carrot, grated
1 cup crushed, fresh or canned unsweetened pineapple
2 tablespoons currants
1 tablespoon toasted sesame seeds
1 cup Tartare Sauce (see p. 113)

Thoroughly combine all ingredients. Spoon into a glass salad bowl. Chill and serve.

Lettuce and fruit salad

SERVES 4

2 bananas, sliced
3 kiwi fruit, peeled and sliced
1 orange, peeled and segmented
1 salad bowl filled with lettuce, endive and mignonette pieces (bite-size)
1 cup Tangy Yoghurt Dressing (see p. 113)

Carefully combine fruit and spoon into bowl of lettuce pieces. Spoon Tangy Yoghurt Dressing over the salad.

Mushroom salad

SERVES 4

2 Spanish onions, thinly sliced into rings
1 clove garlic, minced
½ red capsicum, seeded and chopped
1 cup Sweet Dressing (see p. 112)
1 tablespoon poppy seeds
10 button mushrooms, halved
chopped parsley for garnishing

Sauté onions, garlic, capsicum and Sweet Dressing in an uncovered non-stick pan for about 5 minutes only. Add poppy seeds to the mixture and pour this over the mushrooms. Gently toss to coat mushrooms. Chill and serve with a garnish of chopped parsley.

Potato salad

SERVES 4-6

10 small new potatoes, cooked, peeled and halved
1 small salad onion, finely chopped
1 teaspoon seeds
1½ cups Herb and Yoghurt Dressing (see p. 107)

Arrange potatoes in a wooden bowl. Combine remaining ingredients (seeds such as sesame, poppy, mustard or celery would be
suitable) and spoon over potatoes. Gently toss. Chill and serve.

Orange salad

SERVES 4

4 oranges, peeled
1 salad onion, thinly sliced
1 red capsicum, seeded and chopped
1 green capsicum, seeded and chopped
1 stalk celery, finely diced
½ cup Sweet Dressing (see p. 112)

Segment oranges and remove pith. Then combine all ingredients.
Chill and serve.

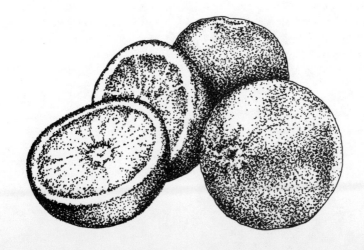

Tomato with capers salad

SERVES 4-6

4 tomatoes, finely sliced
2 tablespoons chopped capers
½ quantity Cucumber Dressing (see p. 106)
sprigs mint for garnishing

Arrange tomato slices in a glass salad bowl and sprinkle capers over them. Spoon dressing over sliced tomato. Chill and serve garnished with mint.

Yummy carrot salad

SERVES 4

4 carrots, grated
1 cup finely chopped, canned unsweetened or fresh pineapple
⅓ cup currants
1 tablespoon toasted sesame seeds

Combine all ingredients. Chill and serve.

Vegetables and vegetable meals

Brussels sprouts and corn au gratin

SERVES 4

1 onion, chopped
1 clove garlic, minced
1 cup skim milk
1 tablespoon low-salt soy sauce (optional)
¼ cup grated low-fat cheese
pinch cayenne pepper
1 tablespoon cornflour mixed with a little water
20–25 Brussels sprouts, lightly steamed
1½ cups corn kernels, lightly steamed

Topping
½ cup soft breadcrumbs (see p. 24)
2 tablespoons grated lemon rind

Preheat oven to 180°C/375°F.
Sauté onion and garlic in a covered non-stick pan until soft, about 5 minutes. Add skim milk, soy sauce, grated cheese and cayenne pepper. Thicken with cornflour. Place steamed sprouts and corn in an ovenproof dish and pour thickened mixture over them. Top with breadcrumbs and lemon rind and bake in oven for about 15 minutes.

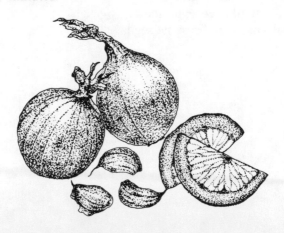

Crispy baked potato shells

SERVES 4

4 large potatoes, steamed

Filling
½ cup dry breadcrumbs (see p. 24)
½ cup unprocessed bran
2 tablespoons snipped chives
1 teaspoon low-salt soy sauce (optional)
½ teaspoon sage or mixed herbs
½ teaspoon garlic powder
pinch cayenne pepper

Preheat oven to 180°C/375°F.
 Halve cooked potatoes and scoop out centre flesh. Combine potato flesh with remaining ingredients and fill each potato centre. Place filled potato halves on a non-stick tray. Bake in oven for about 45 minutes or until crisp. Serve as desired.

VARIATIONS

· The following can be added to the filling.
  1 cup drained canned red kidney beans, soaked for 1 hour in fresh water and drained
  1 cup cooked brown lentils
· Top with tomato slices, cook and serve.
· Garnish with any of the following.
  parmesan cheese, grated
  low-fat hard cheese, grated
  tomato paste and sesame seeds

Crunchy cauliflower

SERVES 4-6

1 cauliflower head, steamed
½ cup water
1 tablespoon low-salt soy sauce (optional)
1 tablespoon skim-milk powder
½ tablespoon cornflour mixed with a little water
pinch garlic powder
pinch powdered ginger
pinch cayenne pepper
¼ cup low-fat grated cheese

Place steamed, heated cauliflower in an oven-proof dish. Combine remaining ingredients except cheese in a small saucepan. Gently simmer, stirring constantly as mixture thickens. Pour over cauliflower, sprinkle with cheese and bake under griller until golden brown.

Curried mixed vegetables

SERVES 4

1 large onion, thinly sliced
4 cloves garlic, minced
½ cup water
1 tablespoon low-salt soy sauce (optional)
1 tablespoon salt-free tomato paste
1½ teaspoons curry powder
pinch powdered ginger
pinch mixed spice
pinch cayenne pepper
4-6 cups steamed fresh or frozen mixed vegetables
2 tomatoes, sliced

Sauté onion and garlic with a little water in a covered non-stick pan. Add remaining water, soy sauce, tomato paste and spices. Stir in steamed vegetables together with tomatoes, heat through and toss. Serve at once.

Fennel and onion braise

SERVES 4

3–4 fennel heads
1 onion, chopped
½ cup vegetable stock
1 tablespoon lemon juice
pinch garlic powder
pinch cayenne pepper

Topping
½ cup soft breadcrumbs (see p. 24)
2 tablespoons grated parmesan cheese

Trim and cut fennel heads into quarters lengthwise. Gently sauté fennel and onion with a little water in a non-stick pan. Add remaining ingredients and gently simmer covered for about 40 minutes or until tender. Top with breadcrumbs and parmesan cheese and bake under griller until golden brown. Serve with roast or as a vegetarian dish.

Hot carrot and potato bake

SERVES 4

4 large potatoes, diced and steamed
4 carrots, diced and steamed
1 tablespoon chopped parsley
¼ cup non-fat, sugar-free yoghurt
1 tablespoon low-salt soy sauce (optional)
1 teaspoon apple juice concentrate
pinch onion powder
pinch garlic powder
pinch cayenne pepper

Topping
2 tablespoons grated low-fat cheese
1 tablespoon oatbran

Sauté potatoes, carrots and parsley in a non-stick pan, tossing as they brown. Spoon into an ovenproof dish. Combine remaining ingredients in pan and heat through, stirring constantly as mixture bubbles. Pour this over vegetable mix. Top with grated cheese and oatbran and bake under griller until golden brown.

VARIATION

Substitute carrots with any of the following suggestions.
1 cup steamed peas
1 cup steamed celery
1 parsnip, diced and steamed
2 cups steamed and diced pumpkin

Potato bean patties

SERVES 4

4 large potatoes
1 small onion, chopped
1 clove garlic, minced
½ cup drained canned red kidney beans
½ teaspoon powdered coriander
pinch cayenne pepper
½ cup unprocessed bran for coating
Hot Chilli Tomato Sauce (see p. 108) for topping

Chop, cook and dry-mash potatoes. Soak red kidney beans in fresh water for 1 hour and drain. Then combine all ingredients and form into small patties. Coat each patty with bran. Brown sides of each patty in a non-stick pan. Serve with a salad and top with Hot Chilli Tomato Sauce.

Sweet potato bake

SERVES 4-6

2 onions, chopped
4 large sweet potatoes, chopped
4 carrots, grated
1 stalk celery, chopped
1 tablespoon low-salt soy sauce (optional)
½ cup canned evaporated skim milk
1½ teaspoons sesame seeds
1 teaspoon cornflour mixed with a little water

Topping
1 cup soft breadcrumbs (see p. 24)
2 tablespoons chopped fresh parsley
1 tablespoon barley bran
1 tablespoon grated parmesan cheese

Preheat oven to 180°C/375°F.
    Sauté onions, sweet potato and grated carrot in a covered non-stick pan until lightly browned. Carefully spoon into an ovenproof dish. Combine remaining ingredients and pour over vegetable mixture. Add topping ingredients and bake in oven for about 40–45 minutes.

Sautéd tomatoes with zucchini

SERVES 4

1 small onion, chopped
4 tablespoons water
4 large tomatoes, sliced
2 zucchini, sliced
1 tablespoon low-salt soy sauce (optional)
1 teaspoon apple juice concentrate
pinch garlic powder
pinch powdered ginger
pinch cayenne pepper

Sauté onion and water in a non-stick pan until tender. Add remaining ingredients and simmer covered for about 10 minutes. Serve as a vegetable or with a roast.

Sautéd snow peas with sesame seeds

SERVES 4

20–25 snow peas
¼ cup water
1 teaspoon chopped mint
1 teaspoon sesame seeds

Sauté all ingredients in an uncovered non-stick pan, gently tossing as peas cook. Remove tips just prior to serving.

Spiced vegetables

SERVES 4

3 potatoes, chopped
4 Brussels sprouts, halved
1 carrot, chopped
1 onion, chopped
1 small sweet potato, chopped
1 small swede, chopped
1 cup water
1 tablespoon low-salt soy sauce (optional)
1 tablespoon cornflour mixed with a little water
1 teaspoon salt-free tomato paste
1 teaspoon garlic powder
½ teaspoon ginger powder
¼ teaspoon chilli powder
pinch cayenne pepper

Steam together all vegetables until just crispy. Combine remaining ingredients with water and pour over steamed vegetables. Gently simmer for about 5 minutes until heated through.

Baked beans on toast

SERVES 4

4 slices toast (see p. 24)
1 × 420 g/15 oz can butter beans
1 cup fat-free, sugar-free commercial pasta sauce
generous pinch cayenne pepper

Soak butter beans in fresh water for 1 hour and drain. Then combine all ingredients in a small uncovered saucepan and heat. Stir occasionally as mixture thickens. Serve with toast.

Baked stuffed zucchini

SERVES 6

6 zucchini, halved lengthwise

Filling
2 onions, chopped
1 small swede, grated
1 clove garlic, minced
1 tablespoon salt-free tomato paste
1 tablespoon low-salt soy sauce (optional)
generous pinch cayenne pepper

Topping
½ cup soft breadcrumbs (see p. 24)
1 teaspoon sesame seeds

Preheat oven to 180°C/375°F.
   Scoop out a small amount of flesh from each zucchini half. Place zucchini lengthwise in an ovenproof dish. Combine filling ingredients with scooped-out flesh from the zucchini and fill each zucchini. Sprinkle with topping ingredients and bake in oven for about 1 hour.

Bean-stuffed capsicum

SERVES 4

2 cups Taco Bean Filling (see p. 68)
2 capsicums, halved lengthwise, seeded

Topping
1 cup soft breadcrumbs (see p. 24)
1 tablespoon oatbran
¼ cup low-fat grated cheese
¼ teaspoon dried, flaked parsley

Preheat oven to 180°C/375°F.
   Divide bean mixture into 4 equal portions. Fill each capsicum half with the mixture and place on an ovenproof tray. Top with breadcrumbs, oatbran, cheese and parsley. Bake in oven for about 15 minutes.

Cheese fingers

SERVES 4

4 slices bread (see p. 24)
4 tablespoons Fruit Chutney (see p. 102)
½ cup grated low-fat cheese
1 tablespoon sesame seeds

Spread chutney onto face of each slice of bread. Cut into fingers. Top with grated cheese and sesame seeds. Brown under griller.

VARIATION

Add any of the following as a base for the spread.
1 cup steamed chicken pieces with skin and fat removed
185 g/6 oz can water-packed, flaked salmon, drained, skin and
   bones removed
1 cup cooked minced beef, with fat removed
185 g/6 oz can water-packed, flaked tuna, drained
1 spear of canned asparagus onto each finger

Corn and carrot strudel

SERVES ABOUT 4

4 sheets filo pastry

Filling
1 cup steamed corn kernels
1 large potato, boiled and diced
1 large carrot, grated
1 small swede, grated
¼ cup grated low-fat cheese (save half for topping)
1 tablespoon low-salt soy sauce (optional)
½ teaspoon onion powder
½ teaspoon garlic powder
pinch cayenne pepper

Preheat oven to 180°C/375°F.

Combine all filling ingredients. Spread over pastry (4-sheet thickness). Starting at one end, gently roll up pastry. Place on a non-stick tray. Top with remaining cheese and bake for about 40 minutes.

VARIATION

Add ½–1 tablespoon of curry powder to the filling mixture.

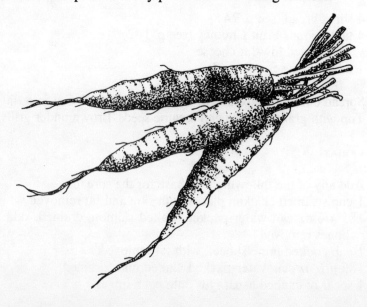

Jack's bean 'n' vegetable stew

SERVES 4

1 × 350 g/12 oz can 4-bean mix
1 onion, chopped
1 clove garlic, crushed
1 carrot, sliced
2 stalks celery, diced
½ green capsicum, seeded and chopped
¼ cup snipped chives
1 cup water
1 tablespoon low-salt soy sauce (optional)
½ teaspoon dried basil
½ teaspoon mixed herbs of choice
generous pinch cayenne pepper

Soak beans in fresh water for 1 hour and then drain. Combine onion, garlic, carrot, celery, capsicum, chives and water in a large saucepan and simmer covered for about 15 minutes. Add remaining ingredients and simmer for a further 5 minutes. Serve with mashed vegetables and salad.

Lentils with mixed rice pilaf

SERVES 4-6

2 onions, chopped
1 tablespoon low-salt soy sauce (optional)
1 teaspoon apple juice concentrate
1 teaspoon garlic powder
1 teaspoon mixed spice
generous pinch cayenne pepper
½ cup cooked brown or green lentils
1½ cups cooked mixed rice (white, brown and wild)

Sauté onions, soy sauce, apple juice concentrate, herbs and spices in a covered non-stick pan until tender. Toss lentils and rice through mixture and serve at once.

Mixed vegie roll-up

SERVES 4

4 sheets filo pastry

Filling
5 cups grated mixed vegetables of choice
½ cup non-fat, salt-free ricotta cheese
1 tablespoon low-salt soy sauce (optional)
1 teaspoon garlic powder
pinch cayenne pepper

Topping
¼ cup oatbran
1 tablespoon grated parmesan cheese

Preheat oven to 180°C/375°F.
   Combine all filling ingredients and spread over filo pastry (4-sheet thickness). Starting at one end, gently roll up pastry. Place on a non-stick tray. Top with oatbran and parmesan cheese. Bake for about 40 minutes.

Capsicum risotto

SERVES 4

1 onion, chopped
1 small red capsicum, seeded and chopped
1 green capsicum, seeded and chopped
1 clove garlic, minced
1 large tomato, chopped
1½ cups cooked mixed rice (white, brown and wild)
1 tablespoon low-salt soy sauce (optional)
½ teaspoon powdered sage
½ teaspoon basil
½ teaspoon oregano
generous pinch cayenne pepper
snipped chives for garnishing

Sauté onion, capsicum, garlic and tomato in a covered non-stick pan for about 5 minutes. Add rice and remaining ingredients, tossing through as they heat. Garnish with chives and serve at once.

Ratatouille

SERVES 4

1 eggplant, diced
1 zucchini, sliced
2 onions, thinly sliced
2 cloves garlic, crushed
3 large tomatoes, quartered
½ green capsicum, seeded and chopped
½ red capsicum, seeded and chopped
½ cup salt-free tomato paste
1 tablespoon low-salt soy sauce (optional)
1 teaspoon apple juice concentrate
generous pinch cayenne pepper

Combine all ingredients in a large saucepan. Gently simmer un-covered until eggplant is tender, about 15 minutes.

Spaghetti sauce

SERVES 4

1 cup chopped, drained canned tomatoes
1 × 500 g/1 lb jar fat-free, sugar-free commercial pasta sauce
1 tablespoon salt-free tomato paste
generous pinch cayenne pepper

Combine all ingredients in a large saucepan. Gently simmer un-covered until heated through. Use as a sauce over cooked egg-yolk-free spaghetti or pasta.

VARIATION

Add about 400 g/14 oz fat-free, minced and cooked topside steak.

Spicy mushroom pasta

SERVES 4

1 quantity egg-yolk-free pasta for 4

Filling
2 cloves garlic, minced
1 red capsicum, seeded and chopped
1 green capsicum, seeded and chopped
32 button mushrooms
½ cup moselle
2 tablespoons low-salt soy sauce (optional)
4 tablespoons chopped parsley
generous pinch cayenne pepper
1 teaspoon grated parmesan cheese for garnishing

Sauté garlic and capsicum in a covered non-stick pan until tender. Add remaining ingredients. Gently simmer covered for about 5 minutes. Serve over heated cooked pasta and top with parmesan cheese.

Sweet-potato crêpes

SERVES 6

6 Plain Crêpes (see p. 98)

Filling
2 cups cooked, dry-mashed sweet potato
½ tablespoon low-salt soy sauce (optional)
½ teaspoon onion powder
½ teaspoon garlic powder
½ teaspoon rosemary
generous pinch cayenne pepper
1 cup Pumpkin and Sesame Seed Sauce (see p. 111)

Keep crêpes warm as you make the filling. Combine filling ingredients. Divide into 6 equal portions. Spoon a portion onto each warmed crêpe and roll up. Serve with heated sauce.

Tomato and chickpea casserole

SERVES 4

1 large onion, sliced
4 cloves garlic, crushed
1 small green capsicum, seeded and chopped
1 cup cooked chickpeas
1 cup fresh or frozen corn kernels
3 cups salt-free tomato juice
4 tablespoons fat-free, sugar-free commercial pasta sauce
1 tablespoon low-salt soy sauce (optional)
½ teaspoon powdered sage
½ teaspoon powdered ginger
generous pinch cayenne pepper

Sauté onion, garlic and capsicum in a covered non-stick pan until tender. Combine with remaining ingredients in a large saucepan. Gently simmer covered for about 15 minutes.

VARIATION

Omit tomato juice and pasta sauce. Add 3 cups defatted stock, 1 cup chopped mushrooms and ½ cup sprouted mung beans (2-day sprouts only). Thicken with 1 tablespoon cornflour.

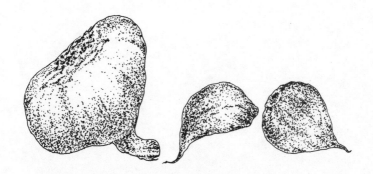

Tacos

SERVES 6-8

6-8 taco shells, warmed

Filling
1 × 400 g/14 oz can red kidney beans
1 × 500 g/1 lb jar fat-free, sugar-free commercial pasta sauce
½ teaspoon chilli powder
generous pinch cayenne pepper

Salad ingredients
2 cups finely chopped lettuce
1 small salad onion, sliced into rings
1 small tomato, thinly sliced
1 small cucumber, thinly sliced

Soak red kidney beans in fresh water for 1 hour and drain. Then combine all filling ingredients in a large saucepan. Gently simmer covered until heated through. Divide mixture into equal portions and fill each taco shell. Top filling of each taco with salad ingredients and serve.

Sandwich fillings

There are a host of delicious fillings that will make superb sandwiches. Here is a small collection from which to choose. If you prefer your sandwich hot, then toast the bread or make sandwich toasts in an electric sandwich-maker. Use only approved breads (see p. 24) and do not use fatty or oily spreads on the bread. Select any of the following fillings or make up your own, but remain within the diet guidelines. Remember, you can liberally use commercial, sugar-free fruit spreads on breads, crêpes, pancakes and toast.

- finely grated apple, natural sultanas, and cinnamon
- drained canned asparagus, non-fat ricotta cheese, and tomato slices
- Baked Beans (see p. 60), grated low-fat cheese, and thinly sliced lettuce
- banana slices, mixed sprouts, and thinly sliced lettuce
- mashed banana, thinly sliced lettuce, and sesame seeds
- thinly sliced cabbage, Fruity Dressing (see p. 106), and mixed sprouts
- thinly sliced cabbage, grated low-fat cheese, and freshly grated beetroot
- chopped celery, non-fat ricotta cheese, and sesame seeds
- Chickpea and Date Spread (see p. 100)
- cucumber slices, tomato slices and shredded lettuce
- hard-boiled egg whites, grated low-fat cheese, and ¼ teaspoon curry powder, all mashed together
- fat-free meat (as per guidelines), Fruit Chutney (see p. 102) and alfalfa sprouts
- finely chopped mushrooms and onion, and mixed sprouts
- natural sultanas, finely chopped celery, and alfalfa sprouts
- tomato slices and finely sliced salad onion soaked in vinegar and then drained
- watercress and thinly sliced cucumber

Meat

Beef olives with mushroom sauce

SERVES 4

8 × 50 g/2 oz thin beef slices
 (about 5 cm × 10 cm/2 in. × 4 in.)
parsley for garnishing

Filling
1 cup of Apple Rice Stuffing (see p. 115)
8 wooden toothpicks

Sauce
2 cups chopped mushrooms
½ green capsicum, seeded and chopped
½ cup white wine
3 tablespoons canned evaporated skim milk
1 tablespoon low-salt soy sauce (optional)
1 tablespoon cornflour mixed with a little water

Remove skin and fat from the meat, roll each piece flat and prepare
stuffing. Divide stuffing into 8 equal portions. Place a portion on
each piece of meat. Roll up and secure with toothpick. Place olives
in a non-stick pan and gently brown on all sides with the lid on
for about 45 minutes until cooked. Set aside and keep hot.
Combine mushrooms and capsicum with liquids in a small
saucepan. Gently simmer covered for about 15 minutes until
tender. Thicken with cornflour and serve over hot beef olives.

Beef steaks

SERVES 4

4 × 100 g/3½ oz fillet steaks

Sauce
1 onion, chopped
1 cup chopped button mushrooms
1 clove garlic, minced
1 cup defatted stock
1 tablespoon salt-free tomato paste
1 tablespoon low-fat soy sauce (optional)
1 teaspoon mixed herbs
generous pinch cayenne pepper

Remove fat from the steaks and cook in a non-stick pan to desired rareness. Set aside and keep hot. Combine sauce ingredients in a non-stick pan and gently simmer for about 15 minutes. Serve sauce over cooked steaks.

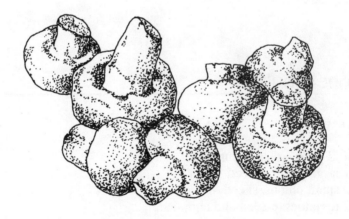

Beef in apple juice

SERVES 4

400 g/14 oz lean round beef
2 onions, sliced
1 clove garlic, minced
1 tablespoon salt-free tomato paste
1½ cups unsweetened apple juice
½ cup water
1 tablespoon low-salt soy sauce (optional)
½ teaspoon oregano
½ teaspoon thyme
generous pinch cayenne pepper
1 bay leaf
½ tablespoon cornflour mixed with a little water

Remove fat and skin from the meat and cut into cubes. Sauté meat, onion and garlic in an uncovered non-stick pan for about 10 minutes. Transfer with tomato paste, liquids, herbs, pepper and bay leaf into a large saucepan. Gently simmer covered for about 1 hour or until meat is tender. Thicken with cornflour, remove bay leaf and serve.

Beef goulash

SERVES 4

400 g/14 oz lean round beef
1 large potato, sliced
2 small onions, sliced
2 tomatoes, peeled and chopped
1 cup water
1 tablespoon low-salt soy sauce (optional)
1 tablespoon apple juice concentrate
1 tablespoon paprika
generous pinch cayenne pepper
¼ cup canned evaporated skim milk
2 tablespoons salt-free tomato paste
paprika for garnishing

Remove skin and fat from the meat and cut into cubes. Place all ingredients except skim milk and tomato paste in a large saucepan. Gently simmer covered for about 45 minutes or until meat is tender. Add remaining ingredients and simmer for a further 10 minutes. Garnish with paprika and serve over cooked egg-yolk-free pasta of choice.

Chilli con carne

SERVES 4

1 × 300 g/10 oz can red kidney beans
400 g/14 oz lean beef
3 onions, sliced
1 clove garlic, crushed
1 × 420 g/15 oz can salt-free tomatoes
1 green capsicum, seeded and chopped
½ cup water
½ cup red wine
1 teaspoon chilli powder
pinch cayenne pepper
1 tablespoon cornflour mixed with a little water

Soak the beans in fresh water for 1 hour, drain and then set aside. Remove skin and fat from the meat and cut into cubes. Sauté meat in a non-stick pan until browned. Add onion, garlic, tomatoes, capsicum, liquids and spices. Gently simmer covered for 1 hour. Add beans and thicken with cornflour about 10 minutes before cooking is completed.

Fruited beef kebabs

SERVES 4

400 g/14 oz lean beef
1 large onion, cut into wedges
1 red capsicum, seeded and cut into 2.5 cm/1 in. pieces
1 banana, cut into 2.5 cm/1 in. pieces
8 × 2.5 cm/1 in. pieces papaw
8 × 2.5 cm/1 in. pieces pineapple
1 teaspoon cornflour mixed with a little water (if necessary)
4 metal skewers

Marinade
1 cup Kebab Marinade (see p. 117)

Remove skin and fat from the meat and cut into 2.5 cm/1 in. cubes. Marinate meat for at least 2 hours, stirring occasionally. Remove meat from marinade and, with other ingredients, thread alternately onto each metal skewer. Wrap each kebab in foil and bake over barbecue for about 5 minutes, turning kebabs every few minutes to prevent burning. Serve over hot, cooked rice. If enough marinade remains, thicken with a little cornflour and serve over kebabs.

VARIATION

Recipe and instructions as above, omitting the beef and using any of the following substitutes, cutting into cubes: lamb, pork, chicken or veal. Meat must be lean.

Quick-to-make hamburgers

SERVES 4

400 g/14 oz lean round beef
¼ cup unprocessed bran
1 teaspoon onion powder
1 teaspoon garlic powder
½ teaspoon curry powder
pinch cayenne pepper
extra unprocessed bran for coating

Remove skin and fat from meat and mince. Thoroughly combine all ingredients and form portions into patties. Coat each patty in bran. Brown each side in a non-stick pan, cooking each side for about 8–10 minutes. Put hamburger in approved roll (see p. 24) with salad of choice.

Sweet roast lamb

100 g / 3 ½ oz PER SERVE

1 × 500 g / 1 lb top-of-leg lamb
1 tablespoon apple juice concentrate
1 tablespoon low-salt soy sauce
1 tablespoon sugar-free commercial apricot spread
1 tablespoon wholemeal flour

Preheat oven to 200°C/400°F.

Remove skin and fat from the meat. Combine all liquids and paint outside of lamb. Lightly dust with the flour. Place meat in an ovenproof dish. Roast covered in oven for about 1 hour or until meat is cooked. Allow to stand for 15 minutes before carving.

VARIATIONS

· Add 1 tablespoon rosemary flakes to flour.
· Replace the lamb with top-of-leg veal.

Curried lamb

SERVES 4

400 g/14 oz trim lamb
1 tablespoon wholemeal plain flour
2–3 teaspoons curry powder
1 onion, chopped
1 clove garlic, minced
1 carrot, sliced into rings
1½ cups water or defatted stock
1 tablespoon salt-free tomato paste
1 tablespoon low-salt soy sauce (optional)
1 tablespoon canned evaporated skim milk
1 tablespoon natural sultanas
½ banana, mashed
generous pinch cayenne pepper

Remove skin and fat from the meat and cut into cubes. Combine flour with 1 teaspoon curry powder and coat the lamb. Place meat, remaining flour mixture, onion, garlic and carrot in a non-stick pan. Dry sauté, carefully tossing as ingredients begin to brown. Place sautéed mixture in a large saucepan with remaining ingredients except curry powder. Simmer covered for about 1 hour or until meat is tender. Add remaining curry powder about 5 minutes before cooking is completed.

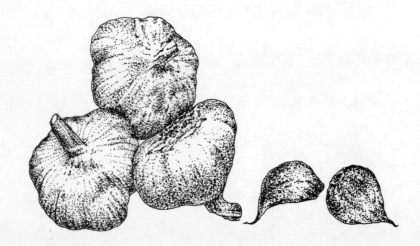

Lamb with mushroom sauce

SERVES 4

4 × 100 g/3½ oz trim lamb butterfly steaks
chopped parsley for garnishing

Sauce
1 large onion, chopped
8 mushrooms, sliced
½ cup water
3 tablespoons canned evaporated skim milk
1 tablespoon low-salt soy sauce (optional)
1 teaspoon apple juice concentrate
pinch cayenne pepper
1 tablespoon cornflour mixed with a little water

Remove skin and fat from the steaks. Place steaks in a large non-stick pan and sauté both sides until cooked to desired consistency (some like it pink). Set aside and keep hot. Combine ingredients for the sauce, except cornflour, in a small saucepan. Simmer covered for about 15 minutes or until onion is tender. Thicken with cornflour and serve over cooked lamb steaks. Garnish with parsley.

Braised veal chops with prunes

SERVES 4

4 × 100 g/3½ oz veal chops
1 large onion, sliced into rings
2 stalks celery, sliced diagonally
12 prunes, pitted
1 bay leaf
3 tablespoons salt-free tomato paste
1 cup water
¼ cup moselle
1 tablespoon low-salt soy sauce (optional)
1 tablespoon cornflour mixed with a little water
¼ teaspoon dried sage
pinch cayenne pepper

Remove fat from the veal chops. Gently sauté chops in an un-covered non-stick pan for about 3 minutes each side. Add onion, celery, prunes, bay leaf and liquids and simmer covered for about 30 minutes. Stir in remaining ingredients about 5 minutes before completion of cooking. Remove bay leaf and serve.

Veal casserole

SERVES 4

400 g/14 oz veal
2 onions, chopped
2 cloves garlic, crushed
2 cups water
1 small carrot, sliced
1 small turnip, cubed
1 tablespoon low-salt soy sauce (optional)
1 teaspoon mixed herbs of choice
generous pinch cayenne pepper
1 tablespoon cornflour mixed with a little water

Remove skin and fat from the veal and cut meat into cubes. Sauté veal, onion, garlic and water in a non-stick pan for about 5 minutes. Add remaining ingredients except cornflour and simmer for a further 40 minutes. Thicken with cornflour and serve.

VARIATIONS

- Add 1 cup sliced mushrooms.
- Add 4 canned salt-free tomatoes, chopped.

Pork kebabs

SERVES 4

4 × 100 g/3½ oz lean pork fillet
1 cup Kebab Marinade using white wine (see p. 117)
1 large onion, quartered and separated
1 apple, cored and cut into pieces
1 green capsicum, seeded and cut into squares
1 teaspoon cornflour mixed with a little water (if necessary)
4 metal skewers

Remove skin and fat from pork. Dice the pork and marinate for at least 4 hours, turning occasionally. Remove meat from marinade and thread alternately with other ingredients onto each metal skewer. Wrap each kebab in foil and bake over barbecue for about 10 minutes, turning kebabs every few minutes to prevent burning. If enough marinade remains, thicken with a little cornflour and serve as a sauce.

Pork casserole with vegetables

SERVES 4

400 g/14 oz lean pork fillet
1 small onion, chopped
1 carrot, diced
½ cup peas
½ cup finely sliced cabbage
1 stalk celery
1 cup water
1 tablespoon skim-milk powder
1 tablespoon low-salt soy sauce (optional)
½ teaspoon apple juice concentrate
pinch cayenne pepper
1 tablespoon cornflour mixed with a little water

Remove skin and fat from the pork and dice it. Place all ingredients except cornflour in a large saucepan. Gently simmer covered for about 1 hour or until meat is tender. Thicken with cornflour and serve.

Roast pork

100 g/3½ oz PER SERVE

500 g/1 lb pork forloin roast
2 tablespoons unprocessed bran
1 tablespoon sesame seeds

Preheat oven to 180°C/375°F.
   Remove skin, fat and bones from meat. Combine bran and sesame seeds and coat outside of pork. Place coated meat in an ovenproof dish and bake, covered, in oven for about 1 hour or until meat is tender.

VARIATION

Rub 2 tablespoons apple juice concentrate to outside of pork before coating with bran and sesame seeds.

Chicken

Chicken with rice

SERVES 4

4 × 100 g/3½ oz chicken breasts
1 onion, chopped
1 clove garlic, minced
½ cup water
1 tablespoon salt-free tomato paste
1 tablespoon low-salt soy sauce (optional)
1 small piece ginger, grated
pinch cayenne pepper
4 cups brown and wild rice cooked with garlic

Remove skin and fat from chicken. Brown each chicken breast on both sides in an uncovered non-stick pan. Set aside and keep hot. Sauté onion, garlic and water in a non-stick covered pan for about 5 minutes. Add remaining ingredients and simmer covered for a further 3 minutes. Add hot chicken breasts and serve over heated rice.

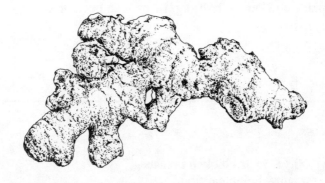

Chicken casserole

SERVES 4

400 g/14 oz chicken fillets
1 onion, chopped
1 clove garlic, crushed
4 tomatoes, chopped
1 potato, diced
1 carrot, diced
1 cup fresh or frozen peas
½ cup fresh or frozen corn kernels
1½ cups water
1 tablespoon low-salt soy sauce (optional)
1 tablespoon cornflour mixed with a little water
½ teaspoon sage
1 bay leaf
pinch cinnamon
pinch cayenne pepper

Remove skin and fat from chicken. Dice chicken and place it together with vegetables and water in a large saucepan. Gently simmer covered for about 40 minutes or until vegetables are tender. Add remaining ingredients about 5 minutes before serving. Remove bay leaf and serve.

VARIATION

Replace chicken with 400 g/14 oz lean beef, diced.

Chicken with a difference

SERVES 4

4 × 100 g/3½ oz chicken breasts
1 teaspoon wholemeal flour
1 teaspoon grated parmesan cheese
1 teaspoon dried parsley

Remove skin and fat from chicken. Combine flour, cheese and sesame seeds in a plastic bag. Lightly coat each chicken breast with the mixture. Place each chicken breast in a non-stick pan and brown each side, allowing about 5 minutes per side until cooked. Serve with vegetables, salad and a gravy chosen from those given on pages 115, 118 and 119.

Pan-fried chicken drumsticks

SERVES 4

4 small chicken drumsticks
1½ cups Mushroom and Tomato Gravy (see p. 118)

Remove skin and fat from the chicken. Place drumsticks in a covered non-stick pan. Gently 'fry' all sides, turning constantly as they cook, about 15–20 minutes. Remove lid about 10 minutes before completion of cooking, to brown. Serve with Mushroom and Tomato Gravy.

Seafood

Garlic prawns

SERVES 4

16 prawns
1 cup skim milk
½ teaspoon low-salt soy sauce (optional)
1 tablespoon cornflour mixed with a little water
1 teaspoon garlic granules
pinch cayenne pepper

Cook, shell, devein and halve the prawns. Combine skim milk with all ingredients, except prawns, in a non-stick pan. Stir constantly as mixture thickens. Fold prawns into the mixture until heated through, about 10 minutes. Serve in individual dishes with small salad chosen from those given on pages 46–52.

VARIATION

Add 1 teaspoon curry powder to the ingredients.

Pan-fried fish

SERVES 4

4 × 100 g/3½ oz pieces lean, white fish fillets
lemon and lime wedges for garnishing

Remove skin from fish. Place fish pieces in a non-stick pan. Gently brown on one side for about 5 minutes. Carefully turn each piece over and brown the other side until cooked. Serve with lemon and lime wedges. This method will provide cooked fish that is a nice colour on the outside.

VARIATION

Coat fish with a small amount of sesame seeds before cooking.

Tuna Florentine

SERVES 4

1 small onion, thinly sliced
1 clove garlic, minced
1 cup drained canned tomatoes
1½ cups fat-free, sugar-free commercial pasta sauce
1½ cups water-packed, drained, canned, flaked tuna
1 quantity cooked, egg-yolk-free pasta
1 pack frozen spinach
1 teaspoon grated parmesan cheese for garnishing

Thaw and drain spinach and heat before serving. Combine onion, garlic, tomatoes and pasta sauce in a large saucepan. Gently simmer covered for about 15 minutes or until onion is tender. Add tuna and simmer for a further 10 minutes until heated through. Fold through heated pasta. Serve over warmed spinach, topped with parmesan cheese.

VARIATION

Replace tuna with 1½ cups water-packed, drained, canned, flaked salmon, skin and bones removed.

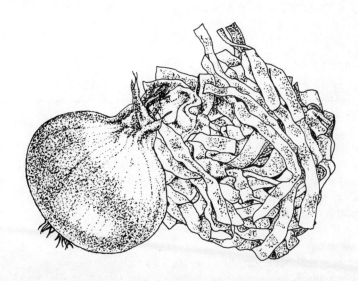

Cakes, desserts and puddings

Apple roly

1 quantity Sweet Pastry (see p. 99)

Filling
1½ cups peeled, cored and sliced apple
½ cup natural sultanas
¼ cup apple juice concentrate
1 tablespoon grated lemon rind

Topping
1 tablespoon apple juice concentrate
1 tablespoon grated lemon peel

Preheat oven to 180°C/375°F.
Roll out pastry into a 26 cm/10 in. square. Combine apple, sultanas, apple juice concentrate and grated lemon rind. Spread apple mixture over surface of pastry. Roll up to form a log. Carefully place on a non-stick tray. Mix remaining apple juice concentrate with lemon peel and sprinkle over pastry log. Bake in oven for about 20 minutes.

Apricot crumble

SERVES 4-6

1 × 800 g/1¾ lb canned apricots in natural juice, drained
1 quantity Sweet Mincemeat (see p. 104)
1 teaspoon nutmeg
pinch cinnamon

Topping
½ cup soft breadcrumbs (see p. 24)
1 teaspoon sesame seeds

Preheat oven to 200°C/400°F.

Arrange apricot halves, outside uppermost, in a round, oven-proof dish. Combine Sweet Mincemeat and spices and spread over apricots. Sprinkle breadcrumbs and sesame seeds on top. Bake in oven for about 30 minutes.

Baked fruit apples

SERVES 4

4 green apples, cored
4 tablespoons Sweet Mincemeat (see p. 104)
½ cup fresh orange juice
½ teaspoon cinnamon

Preheat oven to 180°C/375°F.

Fill the centre of each apple with the Sweet Mincemeat. Place on a non-stick tray. Pour orange juice over the apples and dust with cinnamon. Bake in oven for about 1 hour or until cooked.

Fruit cake citrus

1 cup pitted and chopped dates
½ cup natural sultanas
¼ cup brandy
½ cup fresh orange juice
½ cup fresh lemon juice
2 cups wholemeal self-raising flour
¼ cup ricebran granules
1 egg white
1 teaspoon mixed spice
¼ teaspoon powdered ginger

Preheat oven to 200°C/400°F.

Soak fruit, brandy and juices overnight. Next day combine all ingredients. Spoon into a 20 cm/8 oz tin lined with non-stick baking paper. Bake for about 30 minutes then reduce oven temperature to 170°C/325°F and bake for 1 hour or until cooked. Cool in airtight tin.

Peaches with creamed rice

SERVES 4

¾ cup white rice
¼ cup brown rice
about 1½ cups skim milk
¼ cup apple juice concentrate
¼ teaspoon lemon juice
1 teaspoon grated lemon rind
4 canned peach halves, diced
extra skim milk (if necessary)
grated nutmeg for garnishing

Cook white and brown rice with skim milk until soft, adding extra skim milk if necessary. Cool. Add apple concentrate, lemon juice and rind. Gently fold peaches through rice. Spoon into individual dishes and garnish with nutmeg. Chill and serve.

VARIATION

Replace peaches with 1–2 cups unsweetened fruit salad.

Fruit loaf

1 cup raisins
1 teaspoon allspice
pinch cinnamon
1 cup skim milk
1 cup freshly grated beetroot
1½ cups wholemeal self-raising flour
2 egg whites, stiffly beaten
2 tablespoons apple juice concentrate

Preheat oven to 200°C/375°F.
    Soak raisins and spices with a little skim milk overnight. Next day combine all ingredients and thoroughly mix. Spoon mixture into a loaf tin lined with non-stick baking paper. Bake in oven for about 45 minutes. Cool in an airtight tin.

VARIATION

Replace raisins with 1 cup natural sultanas.

Topping suggestions
· sesame seeds, toasted
· poppy seeds
· mixed orange and lemon peel
· dried fruit, puréed

Old-fashioned steamed pudding

1 cup pitted and chopped dates
½ cup natural sultanas
1 cup fresh orange juice
1½ cups wholemeal self-raising flour
1 teaspoon cinnamon
grated orange rind

Soak fruit in orange juice overnight. Next day combine all ingredients and thoroughly mix. Spoon into a small steamer, seal and place in a saucepan of water. Gently simmer for about 1½ hours, making sure there is sufficient water in saucepan.

VARIATION

Add ½ cup chopped, drained canned chickpeas.

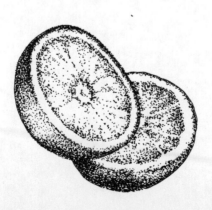

Simple-to-make pudding

SERVES 4

1 large Plain Pancake (see p. 99), freshly made
4 tablespoons commercial strawberry spread
1 punnet washed and hulled strawberries, saving 4 for garnishing
1 tablespoon apple juice concentrate
½ teaspoon cinnamon
1½ cups Tangy Yoghurt Dressing (see p. 113)

Spread strawberry spread onto hot pancake. Combine strawberries, apple concentrate and cinnamon. Arrange coated fruit on
top of spread. Cut pancake into four. Place each portion on a flat
dish. Cover with Tangy Yoghurt Dressing (either warmed or cold)
and garnish with one strawberry.

Fruit desserts and whips

Fruit sauces

The range of sauces that can be served with hot or cold desserts
and puddings is enormous. Here are some suggestions you might
like to use in place of sauces that have a heavy skim-milk base.
- strawberries, with apple juice concentrate or alone
- blueberries, frozen; thaw and mix with orange juice
- mango and papaw with unsweetened pineapple juice
- pears with passionfruit pulp
- banana with orange juice and cinnamon
- pears with fresh ginger
- pineapple and pear with cinnamon
- papaw with pineapple

Purée fruit or mixed fruits of choice in a blender. Serve chilled,
warmed or at room temperature. For extra dash, add 1 tablespoon
chopped, drained canned chickpeas.

Fresh mango salad

SERVES 4

4 mangoes, peeled and diced
pulp 6 passionfruit
1 cup pear and ginger sauce (see above)

Gently combine mangoes with passionfruit pulp. Spoon into individual glass dishes. Chill and serve with pear and ginger sauce.

Frozen fruit dessert

SERVES 4

4 small bananas
2 cups washed and hulled strawberries
pulp 6 passionfruit

Freeze bananas in their skins until hard. Carefully peel and place in blender with strawberries. Purée until mixture thickens. Fold in passionfruit. Spoon into a container and freeze. Use on its own or over your favourite dessert.

Frozen fruits

MAKES ABOUT 3 CUPS

½ pineapple, well ripened
1 apple, cored and chopped
1 pear, chopped
pulp 4 passionfruit (optional)

Purée all ingredients except passionfruit pulp. Fold in passionfruit pulp. Pour into individual ice-cube containers and freeze. Eat as a frozen dessert or as ice-cubes.

Hot breakfast fruit compote

SERVES 4

1 cup pitted prunes
½ cup pitted and chopped dates
¼ cup natural sultanas
¼ cup raisins
4 dried apricots, snipped
1 tablespoon grated lemon rind
1 cup fresh orange juice

Soak fruit, including lemond rind, with orange juice overnight.
Next day heat mixture in a non-stick pan. Serve as a dessert with
non-fat yoghurt or as a breakfast.

Hot winter fruit salad

SERVES 4

1 cup fresh or canned unsweetened pineapple pieces
1 green apple, cored and chopped
1 pear, peeled, cored and chopped
1 orange, peeled, pith removed and chopped
1 nectarine, peeled, pith removed and chopped
1 cup seedless grapes
½ cup fresh or frozen blueberries
½ cup unsweetened grape juice
4–5 cloves
¼ teaspoon cinnamon

Place all ingredients in a large saucepan. Gently warm through
and simmer uncovered for about 5 minutes. Remove cloves. Serve
with non-fat yoghurt.

Strawberry ricotta filling

1 cup non-fat, salt-free ricotta cheese
1 punnet washed and hulled strawberries
¼ cup apple juice concentrate

Purée all ingredients in a blender until smooth. Use as a filling
for pancakes or cheesecake.

VARIATION

Use any of the following fruit as alternative to the strawberries
and apple juice concentrate: dried banana, soaked in water, then
chopped; fresh or frozen blueberries; lemon rind and juice; canned
mandarins; fresh mango; fresh or canned unsweetened pineapple;
passionfruit pulp.

Sauced banana and grapes

SERVES 4

1 teaspoon apple juice concentrate
1 tablespoon Cointreau (optional)
4 bananas, sliced
4 cups seedless grapes
1 cup fresh fruit sauce (see p. 91)

Combine apple concentrate and Cointreau. Mix with bananas and grapes. Spoon into a glass dish. Chill and serve with fruit sauce of choice.

Stuffed fresh nectarines

SERVES 4

4 nectarines, fresh, halved and stoned
½ cup Frozen Fruit Dessert (see p. 92)
1 teaspoon poppy seeds

Prepare nectarines and arrange on a large, round platter. Fill a forcer bag with Frozen Fruit Dessert. Using a star nozzle, squeeze a large star onto the centre of each nectarine half. Sprinkle with seeds and serve at once.

VARIATION

Replace the nectarines with 4 canned unsweetened pineapple rings.

Tipsy oranges

SERVES 4

6 sweet oranges, peeled, pith removed and sliced
¼ cup apple juice concentrate
¼ cup water
¼ cup brandy
2 tablespoons toasted sesame seeds
1 tablespoon grated orange rind

Arrange orange slices in layers in a glass dish. Combine liquids and heat through in a small saucepan. Pour over oranges. Top with sesame seeds and orange rind. Chill for several hours until liquid has soaked through oranges.

Tropical fruits

SERVES 4-6

2 cups diced papaw
1 cup chopped pineapple
1 cup chopped custard apple
1 mango, diced
¼ honeydew melon, diced
1 cup unsweetened pineapple juice
1 large bunch black grapes, off the stem, for garnishing

Combine all ingredients in a large bowl. Top with black grapes. Chill and serve.

VARIATION

Replace black grapes with any of the following: sliced banana, blueberries, sliced kiwi fruit, hulled and halved strawberries.

Pancakes, muffins, crêpes and scones

Buckwheat pancakes

MAKES ABOUT 6

½ cup buckwheat flour
½ cup wholemeal self-raising flour
2 egg whites, stiffly beaten
1 cup skim milk

Combine all ingredients to make a smooth batter. Place 2–3 spoonfuls of mixture into a non-stick pan. Heat through and flip over to cook other side. Repeat with remainder of mixture.

Carrot muffins

MAKES ABOUT 12 MUFFINS

½ cup pitted and chopped dates
½ cup dark, unsweetened grape juice
3 cups grated carrot
¼ cup canned evaporated skim milk
1½ cups wholemeal self-raising flour
¼ cup unprocessed bran
1 egg white
1 cup water
¼ teaspoon cinnamon
good pinch grated nutmeg
good pinch ground ginger

Preheat oven to 200°C/400°F.

Place dates with grape juice in a small saucepan. Gently simmer uncovered for about 5 minutes. Set aside and cool. Combine with remaining ingredients except water. Slowly add water, thoroughly mixing until the mixture is the consistency of a cake mixture. Spoon into non-stick muffin tins. Bake for about 15 minutes or until cooked.

Cheese and herb scones

MAKES ABOUT 8

2 cups wholemeal self-raising flour
1 tablespoon unprocessed bran
2 tablespoons grated low-fat cheese
about ½ cup water
¼ cup canned evaporated skim milk
1 teaspoon mixed herbs
generous pinch cayenne pepper
extra wholemeal self-raising flour for shaping scones

Preheat oven to 220°C/440°F.

Combine all ingredients to make a soft dough. Add extra liquid if necessary. Turn dough onto a well-floured board and form into a large round scone. Cut into rounds and place on a non-stick tray. Bake for about 12 minutes. Cool in an airtight tin.

VARIATION

Omit the herbs and add ¼ cup dry-mashed pumpkin plus 4 extra tablespoons wholemeal self-raising flour.

Currant scones

MAKES ABOUT 8

2 cups wholemeal self-raising flour
½ cup currants
2 tablespoons apple juice concentrate
pinch mixed spice
about 1 cup buttermilk
extra wholemeal self-raising flour for dusting

Preheat oven to 220°C/440°F.

Place flour, currants, apple concentrate and mixed spice in a mixing bowl. Gradually add buttermilk to make a soft dough. Add extra liquid if necessary. Turn dough onto a well-floured board and form into a large round scone. Cut into rounds and place on a non-stick tray. Bake for about 12 minutes. Cool in an airtight tin.

Plain crêpes

MAKES ABOUT 6

1 cup unbleached self-raising flour
2 egg whites, stiffly beaten
1½ cups skim milk

Combine all ingredients in a mixing bowl to make a smooth batter of pouring consistency. Pour ¼ cup of batter onto a non-stick pan. When bubbles appear, flip over to cook other side. Repeat with remaining mixture.

Plain pancakes

MAKES ABOUT 8

¾ cup unbleached self-raising flour
¼ cup unprocessed bran
2 egg whites, stiffly beaten

Combine all ingredients to make a smooth batter. Place spoonfuls onto a non-stick pan. Heat through and flip over to cover other side. Repeat with remaining mixture.

VARIATIONS

- Add 1 cup steamed and diced mixed vegetables of choice plus 1 tablespoon low-salt soy sauce (optional).
- Add 1 cup chopped, drained canned fruit of choice (e.g. peaches, apricots), plus 2 tablespoons apple concentrate.

Sweet pastry

1 cup wholemeal self-raising flour
½ cup unbleached self-raising flour
1 tablespoon ricebran granules
1 tablespoon apple juice concentrate
about ¼ cup water
extra unbleached self-raising flour for dusting

Place all ingredients into a large bowl and carefully stir to make a dough consistency. Add extra water if necessary. Lightly knead and roll out pastry on a well-floured board. Use as desired.

Chutneys, spreads and dips

Apricot chutney

MAKES 3-4 CUPS

20 dried apricots, chopped
1 onion, chopped
1 cup water
3 tomatoes, peeled and chopped
½ cup apple juice concentrate
4 tablespoons salt-free tomato paste
1 cup cider vinegar
1 tablespoon grated fresh ginger
1 teaspoon mustard
generous pinch cayenne pepper

Combine apricots, onion and water in a large saucepan. Gently simmer covered for about 15 minutes. Add remaining ingredients and gently simmer uncovered until mixture is thick, about 40 minutes. Pour into sterilised jars and refrigerate.

Chickpea and date spread

MAKES ABOUT 1½ CUPS

1 cup drained canned chickpeas
¼ cup pitted and chopped dates
¼ cup unsweetened orange juice
1 tablespoon lemon juice
1 tablespoon grated lemon rind

Purée all ingredients in a blender until mixture resembles a smooth spread. Add extra liquid if necessary. Store in refrigerator.

VARIATION

Replace the dates with ¼ cup Sweet Mincemeat (see p. 104).

Plum and raspberry spread

MAKES ABOUT 2 CUPS

10 fresh plums
1 punnet washed and hulled raspberries
¼ cup apple juice concentrate

Place all ingredients in a small saucepan. Slowly bring to boil, covered. Gently simmer for about 1 hour until mixture is thick. Cool and place in sterilised jars. Store in refrigerator.

VARIATION

Replace raspberries with 1 punnet washed and hulled blackberries.

Dried peach spread

MAKES ABOUT 1-1½ CUPS

1 cup chopped dried peaches
½ cup water
¼ cup apple juice concentrate

Soak peaches in water overnight. Next day combine with remaining ingredients in a saucepan and gently simmer covered for about 20 minutes. Cool and purée in a blender. Place in sterilised jars. Store in refrigerator.

VARIATION

Add 1 cup fresh or canned pineapple pieces to the mixture.

Fruit chutney

MAKES ABOUT 3 CUPS

3 tablespoons candied fruit of choice
2 cups chopped mixed dried fruit
½ cup chopped natural sultanas
½ cup unsweetened orange juice
1 cup white vinegar
4 cloves
½ teaspoon cinnamon
½ teaspoon garlic powder
½ teaspoon powdered ginger
½ teaspoon coriander
generous pinch cayenne pepper

Wash, soak and drain the candied fruit. Soak all fruit with orange juice overnight. Next day place soaked fruit in a large saucepan and gently simmer covered for about 15 minutes. Add remaining ingredients, stirring gently. Simmer uncovered for a further 40 minutes, taking care not to burn chutney. Cool and spoon into sterilised jars. Store in refrigerator. Serve with cold meats or hot spicy meats over rice.

Mixed fruit relish

MAKES ABOUT 3 CUPS

8 dried figs, washed and chopped
6 dried apricots, chopped
2 apples, cored, peeled and finely chopped
¼ cup natural sultanas
2 tablespoons currants
1 onion, finely chopped
¼ cup apple juice concentrate
3 tablespoons salt-free tomato paste
1 cup cider vinegar
½ tablespoon mustard seeds
¼ teaspoon cinnamon
generous pinch cayenne pepper

Place all ingredients in a large saucepan. Slowly bring to boil and gently simmer uncovered for about 1 hour or until thick. Spoon into sterilised jars and refrigerate.

Spinach dip

MAKES ABOUT 2 CUPS

1 pack frozen spinach, thawed and drained
1 cup non-fat, salt-free ricotta cheese
2 cloves garlic, crushed
1 tablespoon low-salt soy sauce (optional)
½ cup parsley
1 tablespoon lemon juice
generous pinch cayenne pepper

Purée together all ingredients until smooth. Add extra cayenne pepper if necessary. Chill for about 2–4 hours. Serve with raw vegetables of choice or as a filling in stuffed vegetables.

VARIATIONS

· Replace spinach with 1 cup chopped cooked chicken breast with skin and fat removed.
· Replace spinach with 1 cup cooked and shelled prawns or shrimp.

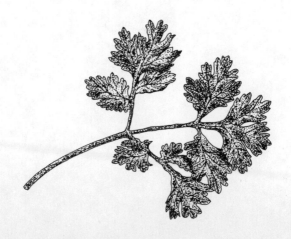

Sweet mincemeat

MAKES ABOUT 2 CUPS

1 cup natural sultanas
1 cup pitted and chopped dates
½ cup mixed orange and lemon peel
1½ cups water
¼ cup lemon juice
2 teaspoons cinnamon
1 teaspoon mixed spice
¼ teaspoon powdered ginger
¼ teaspoon ground cloves
1 tablespoon grated lemon rind

Place all ingredients in a large saucepan. Gently simmer covered until mixture thickens. Spoon into a large, covered container and refrigerate. Use as a spread on approved bread or toast (see p. 24), scones or as a pie or fruit filling for tarts.

Dressings and sauces

Bean sauce

MAKES ABOUT 5 CUPS

1 × 750 g/1½ lb canned red kidney beans
1 × 500 g/1 lb jar fat-free, sugar-free commercial pasta sauce
¼ cup moselle
dash tabasco sauce

Soak beans in fresh water for 1 hour, then drain. Combine all ingredients in a large saucepan. Gently simmer uncovered for about 10 minutes.

Creamy mushroom sauce

MAKES ABOUT 2 CUPS

8 button mushrooms, sliced
1 onion, minced
1½ cups defatted stock
1 tablespoon skim-milk powder
1 tablespoon low-salt soy sauce (optional)
1 tablespoon arrowroot mixed with a little water
¼ teaspoon dry mustard
pinch cayenne pepper

Place mushrooms, onion and stock in a small saucepan. Gently simmer covered for 10 minutes. Add remaining ingredients and thicken with arrowroot.

Cucumber dressing

MAKES ABOUT 2 CUPS

1 cup non-fat, sugar-free yoghurt
½ cucumber, finely chopped
½ small salad onion, finely chopped
½ teaspoon chopped green chilli
chopped parsley for garnishing

Combine all ingredients and serve garnished with parsley. Use as a dressing on salad of choice.

Fruity dressing

MAKES ABOUT 1 CUP

½ cup non-fat, sugar-free yoghurt
½ cup unsweetened pineapple juice
1 tablespoon apple juice concentrate
1 tablespoon chopped parsley
1 tablespoon lemon juice
1 teaspoon mustard

Combine all ingredients. Chill and serve with salad of choice.

Green dressing

MAKES ABOUT 1½ CUPS

1 cup non-fat, sugar-free yoghurt
¼ cup chopped parsley
2 tablespoons chopped mint
2 tablespoons snipped chives
1 tablespoon apple juice concentrate
1 teaspoon mustard
juice 1 lemon
1 tablespoon grated lemon rind

Combine all ingredients. Chill and serve with salad of choice.

Herb and yoghurt dressing

MAKES ABOUT 1½ CUPS

1½ cups non-fat, sugar-free yoghurt
1 tablespoon lemon juice
1 teaspoon dried herbs of choice
pinch cayenne pepper

Dried herbs from which to choose include chives, mint, parsley, basil and sage. Combine all ingredients. Chill and serve with salad of choice.

VARIATION

Add 3 tablespoons apple juice concentrate to the ingredients.

Horseradish sauce

MAKES ABOUT ½ CUP

1½ tablespoons finely grated horseradish
1 tablespoon apple juice concentrate
1 tablespoon vinegar
1 tablespoon canned evaporated skim milk
1 teaspoon low-salt soy sauce (optional)
1 teaspoon dry mustard
pinch cayenne pepper

Combine all ingredients. Chill and serve with your favourite meat.

Hot chilli tomato sauce

MAKES ABOUT 2 CUPS

1 onion, chopped
2 cloves garlic, chopped
1 × 420 g/15 oz can tomatoes, drained and chopped
1 green capsicum, seeded and chopped
1–2 small chilli peppers, chopped
½ teaspoon oregano
generous pinch cayenne pepper

Sauté onion and garlic in a covered non-stick pan until tender, about 5 minutes. Add remaining ingredients and heat through. Purée in a blender until smooth. Serve over tacos or meat of choice. Store in refrigerator.

Hot sauce

SERVES 4-6

2 small onions, chopped
1 clove garlic, minced
1 × 400 g/14 oz can pimientos, drained and chopped
¼ cup salt-free tomato paste
½ cup dry white wine
½ cup water
1 tablespoon low-salt soy sauce (optional)
pinch cayenne pepper

Sauté onion and garlic in non-stick pan until tender. Add remaining ingredients and simmer for a further 5 minutes until sauce thickens. Serve over dry-baked potatoes or meat of choice.

Mint sauce

MAKES ABOUT ½ CUP

6 tablespoons freshly chopped mint
2 tablespoons apple juice concentrate
6 tablespoons vinegar
4 tablespoons hot water

Combine all ingredients and serve over roast lamb.

Minted mango sauce

MAKES ABOUT 1 CUP

1 mango, peeled and chopped
¼ cup drained canned chickpeas
2 tablespoons apple juice concentrate
2 tablespoons chopped mint

Purée together all ingredients in a blender until smooth. Serve over your favourite meat or salad.

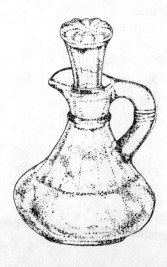

Orange soy dressing

MAKES ABOUT ½ CUP

½ cup unsweetened orange juice
½ clove garlic, crushed
1 small chilli, finely chopped
1 tablespoon chopped parsley
2 tablespoons low-salt soy sauce
2 tablespoons lemon juice
1 tablespoon apple juice concentrate
1 tablespoon grated orange rind

Combine all ingredients together. Chill and serve.

Prune and yoghurt sauce

MAKES ABOUT 2 CUPS

½ cup pitted and chopped prunes
¼ cup water
1½ cups non-fat, sugar-free yoghurt
1 tablespoon apple juice concentrate
1 tablespoon lemon juice
1 tablespoon grated lemon rind

Soak prunes in the water overnight. Next day cook soaked prunes,
apple juice concentrate, lemon juice and rind in a small saucepan.
Purée in a blender with the yoghurt. Chill and serve with salads
or desserts of choice.

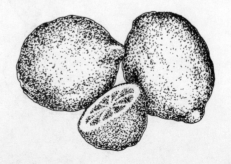

Pumpkin and sesame seed sauce

MAKES ABOUT 1 CUP

2 cups steamed and dry-mashed pumpkin
½ cup defatted stock
1 tablespoon low-salt soy sauce (optional)
½ tablespoon apple juice concentrate
1 tablespoon toasted sesame seeds

Combine mashed pumpkin with remaining ingredients. Heat through in a small saucepan. Serve as a gravy over savoury crêpes or meats of choice.

Rum sauce

MAKES ABOUT 2 CUPS

2 cups non-fat, salt-free ricotta cheese
¼ cup water
¼ cup apple juice concentrate
1 tablespoon rum

Purée together all ingredients in a blender until smooth. Chill and serve with fruit or dessert of choice. If mixture thickens add a little extra water and whip again.

Strawberry dressing

MAKES ABOUT 1 CUP

1 punnet washed and hulled strawberries
1 clove garlic, chopped
¼ cup cider vinegar
2 tablespoons apple juice concentrate
1 tablespoon lemon or lime juice
¼ teaspoon dried oregano
pinch cayenne pepper

Purée together all ingredients in a blender until smooth. Chill and serve over salad of choice.

VARIATION

Replace strawberries with 1 punnet blueberries.

Sweet dressing

MAKES ABOUT 1 CUP

½ clove garlic, crushed
½ cup apple juice concentrate
1 tablespoon lemon juice
½ tablespoon low-salt soy sauce (optional)
pinch cayenne pepper

Combine all ingredients. Chill and serve.

Tangy yoghurt dressing

MAKES ABOUT 1½ CUPS

1½ cups non-fat, sugar-free yoghurt
1 tablespoon apple juice concentrate
½ teaspoon low-salt soy sauce (optional)
1 teaspoon freshly grated ginger
½ teaspoon powdered ginger
1 teaspoon grated orange rind

Combine all ingredients. Chill and serve with fruit or fruit salads.

Tartare sauce

MAKES ABOUT ½ CUP

1 tablespoon apple juice concentrate
1 tablespoon vinegar
1 tablespoon lemon juice
½ tablespoon low-salt soy sauce (optional)
½ small gherkin, finely chopped
2 teaspoons chopped capers
2 teaspoons chopped parsley
½ cup non-fat, sugar-free yoghurt
½ teaspoon mustard
pinch cayenne pepper

Combine all liquids and thoroughly mix. Carefully fold in remaining ingredients. Chill and serve with salad or fish.

Yoghurt mint dressing

MAKES ABOUT 1 CUP

1 cup non-fat, sugar-free yoghurt
3 tablespoons finely chopped mint
2 tablespoons apple juice concentrate
2 tablespoons lemon juice
½ teaspoon paprika
1 tablespoon grated lemon rind
pinch cayenne pepper

Combine all ingredients. Chill in refrigerator and serve over salad of choice.

VARIATION

Replace lemon juice and rind with ¼ cup orange juice and 1 tablespoon grated orange rind.

Gravies, stuffings and marinades

Apple rice stuffing

MAKES ABOUT 2½ CUPS

1 cup cooked brown rice
¼ cup soft breadcrumbs (see p. 24)
1 apple, cored and chopped
1 small onion, chopped
¼ cup defatted stock
1 teaspoon garlic powder
¼ teaspoon mixed dried herbs of choice

Combine all ingredients. Fill cavity of meat of choice, e.g. beef, lamb or pork pockets, whole fish cavity or halved chicken breasts.

VARIATION

Replace apple with 2 canned peach halves.

Apricot and chive gravy

MAKES ABOUT 1½ CUPS

1 cup drained, puréed, canned unsweetened apricots
1 tablespoon snipped chives
½ cup defatted stock
½ tablespoon low-salt soy sauce (optional)
1 tablespoon arrowroot mixed with a little water
pinch garlic powder
pinch cayenne pepper

Combine all ingredients in a small saucepan. Gently heat through, stirring constantly as mixture thickens.

Apricot stuffing

MAKES ABOUT 1¼ CUPS

8 dried apricots, finely snipped
1 onion, chopped
1 cup soft breadcrumbs (see p. 24)
1 egg white
1 tablespoon chopped parsley
½ teaspoon garlic powder
pinch cayenne pepper

Combine all ingredients. Recommended for lamb.

Garlic and rosemary stuffing

MAKES ABOUT 1 CUP

1 cup soft breadcrumbs (see p. 24)
3 large cloves garlic, minced
2 teaspoons dried rosemary
1 tablespoon red wine
pinch cayenne pepper

Combine all ingredients. Recommended for lamb, beef or pork.

Hawaiian marinade

MAKES ABOUT 1¼ CUPS

1 cup unsweetened pineapple juice
1 tablespoon low-salt soy sauce (optional)
1 tablespoon sherry
1 tablespoon apple juice concentrate
1 teaspoon powdered ginger
½ teaspoon garlic granules
½ teaspoon curry powder
generous pinch cayenne pepper

Combine all ingredients. Use to marinate meat of choice, leaving in refrigerator for at least 1 hour.

Hawaiian stuffing

MAKES ABOUT 1 CUP

⅓ cup cooked mixed rice
¼ cup soft breadcrumbs (see p. 24)
1 small ripe banana
1 egg white
½ teaspoon grated fresh ginger
¼ teaspoon dried dill
¼ teaspoon garlic powder
1 tablespoon grated lemon rind

Combine all ingredients. Fill pocket of meat of choice.

Kebab marinade

MAKES ABOUT 1½ CUPS

1 cup defatted stock
¼ cup red wine
2 cloves garlic, minced
1 tablespoon lemon juice
1 teaspoon dried marjoram
generous pinch cayenne pepper

Combine all ingredients.

VARIATION

Replace red wine with white wine.

Mushroom and tomato gravy

MAKES ABOUT 1½ CUPS

1 large tomato, peeled and chopped
8 button mushrooms, thinly sliced
1 cup defatted stock
1 tablespoon low-salt soy sauce (optional)
1 tablespoon arrowroot mixed with a little water
pinch garlic powder
pinch cayenne pepper

Place tomato, mushrooms and stock in a small saucepan. Gently simmer uncovered for about 10 minutes. Add remaining ingredients and heat through, stirring constantly as mixture thickens.

Standard gravy

MAKES ABOUT 1 CUP

1 cup defatted stock
1 tablespoon low-salt soy sauce (optional)
1 tablespoon cornflour mixed with a little water
pinch cayenne pepper

Combine all ingredients in a small saucepan or open non-stick pan. Gently heat through, stirring constantly as mixture thickens.

Steak marinade

MAKES ABOUT 1 CUP

1 onion, finely chopped
½ cup unsweetened apple juice
¼ cup red wine
¼ teaspoon dried tarragon
¼ teaspoon dried thyme
1 bay leaf
generous pinch cayenne pepper

Combine all ingredients. Marinate beef and leave in refrigerator for an hour.

Wine gravy

MAKES ABOUT 1 CUP

¾ cup defatted stock
¼ cup red or white wine
1 tablespoon low-salt soy sauce (optional)
1 tablespoon arrowroot mixed with a little water
pinch cayenne pepper

Combine all ingredients in a small saucepan or non-stick pan. Gently heat through, stirring constantly as mixture thickens.

VARIATION

Add 2 teaspoons garlic granules and 1 teaspoon herbs of choice.

Glossary

beetroot This root vegetable (known in America as *beet*) has leafy green tops, which are also edible and very nutritious.

biscuit Known in America as *cookie*. The word 'cookie' comes from the Dutch *koekje*, which means 'little cake'. The earliest biscuit-style cakes are thought to date back to 7th-century Persia, one of the first countries to cultivate sugar.

cantaloup This fruit is a variety of rockmelon. It was first cultivated near the city of Cantelupe in Italy in the mid-18th century.

capsicum Known also as *sweet pepper* and *bell pepper* (in America), the capsicum is the fruit of a tropical South American shrub. An excellent source of vitamin C, it also contains vitamin A and small amounts of calcium, phosphorous, iron, thiamin, riboflavin and niacin.

chickpeas Also known as *garbanzo beans*, chickpeas are used extensively in the Mediterranean, India and the Middle East for dishes such as hommos and couscous. They are also found in Spanish stews and Italian minestrone.

cornflour Known in America as *cornstarch*. The first clear recording of separating starch from wheat was by Cato (234–149 BC) when he described soaking wheat for 10 days, draining it and wrapping the soaked grains in a cloth before wringing out the starch, which was used for stiffening clothes.

eggplant Also known as *aubergine*. It is an excellent source of vitamin C and a moderate source of potassium, iron, niacin and folate.

kiwi fruit Also known as *Chinese gooseberries*. This fruit is a native of China, where it grows on the edge of forests in the Yangtze Valley. It is an excellent source of vitamin C.

papaw *Papaya* is its formal name but in Australia it is commonly known as 'papaw'. The American papaw is a separate species and different fruit altogether.

pumpkin Also known as *winter squash*. The pumpkin originated in northern Argentina, near the Andes. It is an excellent source of vitamin A.

scones In America these small quick breads are referred to as *biscuits*.

silverbeet This vegetable (also known as *Swiss chard*) is the oldest type of beet known to be used as a vegetable. The Romans recorded it in the 3rd and 4th centuries BC. It is an excellent source of vitamins A and C and iron.

snow pea Also called *mangetout, sugar pea* and *Chinese pea*. This legume is entirely edible, including the pod; hence its French name *mangetout*, or 'eat it all'.

swede Known in America as *rutabaga*, this versatile root vegetable originated in Europe. It resembles the turnip but has yellow flesh.

sweet potato Also known as the *yam*, but in fact the true yam, although similar to the sweet potato, is not related. There are two varieties of sweet potato: one has red skin with orange flesh; the so-called white sweet potato has yellow skin with yellow flesh.

wholemeal Known in America as *wholewheat*. Wholemeal flour is made from the whole grain and contains the wheat germ, which means it has a higher fibre and nutritional content than white flour.

zucchini Also called *courgette*. Zucchini are an excellent source of vitamin C. The zucchini was first developed in Italy.

Index